Yoga Baby

EXERCISES TO HELP YOU BOND WITH YOUR BABY
PHYSICALLY, EMOTIONALLY, AND SPIRITUALLY

Yoga Baby

DeAnsin Goodson Parker, PH.D.

With Karen W. Bressler

BROADWAY BOOKS *New York*

BROADWAY

YOGA BABY. Copyright © 2000 by DeAnsin Goodson Parker, Ph.D., with Karen W. Bressler.

Broadway Books titles may be purchased for business or promotional use or for special sales. For information, please write to: Special Markets Department, Random House, Inc., 1540 Broadway, New York, NY 10036.

BROADWAY BOOKS and its logo, a letter B bisected on the diagonal, are trademarks of Broadway Books, a division of Random House, Inc.

Visit our Web site at www.broadwaybooks.com

The Library of Congress has established a cataloging-in-publication record for this title.

ISBN 0-7679-0405-2

FIRST EDITION

Illustrated by Wendy Wray
Photographs by Sarah Meriams

Yoga Baby is a trademark of the Goodson Parker Wellness Center

00 01 02 03 04 10 9 8 7 6 5 4 3 2 1

This book is dedicated to all first-time parents who have given birth to their very own little stars and have begun the journey toward helping them shine as brightly as possible. With each shining star, the darkness fades further.

Acknowledgments

I would like to thank everyone who has provided invaluable assistance in bringing this book to fruition. I would like to thank Alan Gelb, for encouraging me; Pam Bernstein, my literary agent, for assisting me in perfecting the book proposal; Diane Terman Felenstein, of the Diane Terman Public Relations firm, for pushing me to move forward; Bernadette Anterola, for all her executive secretarial skill; and Broadway Books editors Tracy Behar and Angela Casey, who made this book so special. I would like to thank all the parents and babies who have participated in the Yoga Baby program at the Center and in the book's preparation.

I would like to thank my son, Damien Parker, and his girlfriend, Aria Tudanger, for their thoughts from the adolescent perspective, and my son for his continual encouragement of my work. I would also like to thank Tom Talley for being there for me.

A special thanks to Alexandra Chaprin, my meditation and yoga teacher, who is also my partner at the Goodson Parker Wellness Center and without whom none of this could have been accomplished.

Contents

Yoga Baby

Introduction

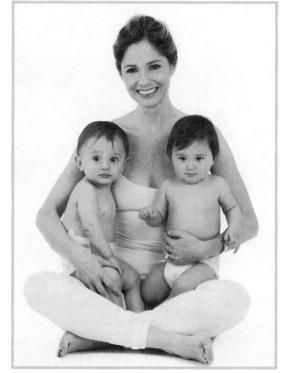

When you and your baby do yoga together, it is about two people getting in harmony so that each feels better connected to the other. What I call "relationship yoga" is an ideal method to learn how to parent intuitively. Relationship yoga is a way to share fun and quality time between parent and baby while building a secure and trusting emotional bond. This is a bond that can be shared throughout your lives. The Yoga Baby™ program is a powerful way to begin this process.

My personal discovery of yoga came at a time when it was the only thing I could turn to for peace and security. It was at this time that I experienced a highly intense personal crisis and desperately needed something to bring me back to a place where I could find balance in my life. The benefits of yoga became quickly apparent to me.

I grew up in a large extended family with grandparents who reached out to all of us in an effort to draw everyone closer together. Their goal was to make sure everyone related to, loved, and supported one another. My grandfather invoked in all of us a sense of generosity of spirit that made our home feel like a bountiful place. At holidays our home was always open to those who had nowhere to go and no one to share the celebration with.

When I was ten years old, my mother became seriously ill and was incapacitated for two years, during which time my father and I took care of my eight-year-old brother, two-year-old sister, and newly born baby sister. I was responsible for cooking the evening meals, keeping up with laundry and housekeeping, caring for my sick mother, and managing my siblings until my father got home from work, all while attending school myself. I also had to support my siblings emotionally when they became anxious about my mother's severe illness, while I constantly feared in my heart that my mother was dying before my very eyes.

As an escape, I would borrow my father's library card and lose myself in reading. Soon I came across a book describing how yoga positions and deep breathing exercises could help relax stressed people. This book changed my life. At first I laughed at the concept and wondered what the big deal was about breathing, especially since I did it every day. I joked about it with my father, who challenged me to try it before forming any conclusions.

I retreated with the book to my room, determined to prove that this breathing routine was ridiculous, only to discover that after just five minutes in a modified lotus position I found myself in a pleasant altered, relaxed state. I was able to breathe more deeply, and I felt less frazzled and impatient. Once I recognized that something significant had happened, I decided to read more. I learned about alternate-nostril breathing, a method that involves breathing in with one nostril and out with the other, and when I tried it, I became aware of how I use my lungs and my chest to breathe.

Despite the fact that I was emotionally spent from caring for my mother, brother, and sisters, these exercises helped me release the tension from my entire body. I remember feeling completely restored within fifteen minutes, sleeping better, and doing better at my schoolwork the next day. I tried pranayama breathing techniques—the practice of conscious breathing through which a yogi is able to gain control over his nervous system or mind. I would lie flat on the floor and go into a meditative state for twenty minutes at a time. Then I experimented with specific yoga postures before I went to sleep. They calmed my anxieties and assured me that I was strong enough to manage and that everything would be fine.

Yet my worry about my mother grew worse. In the stillness of the night after all my chores, I would practice yoga movements, trying to reconnect to my deep inner strength. During those traumatic years, yoga helped me keep it together. I was able to guide my family to leave its strife behind in exchange for peace and connection. We were able to improve our relationships at home, and I began to see a major impact on other areas of my life.

Ultimately, my mother recovered and was able to resume her role in the family. Despite the burdens forced upon us, none of my siblings became emotionally ill or felt neglected throughout our ordeal. We had weathered the storm together and the family stayed whole. Yoga was the force that helped me create that daily union. It has had a very lasting effect, and to this day my family is still incredibly close because of those shared years. I still turn to that spiritual feeling in all aspects of my life to help me align my physical, emotional, mental, and spiritual selves.

Since then, it has been my goal to find ways to share the same beautiful spirit of family with others. Yoga has allowed me to do just that. Through deep breathing, stretching, and certain postures and movements, I was able to discover a relaxed state during which I could open my heart to others. I believe parents should share this magical experience with their children as early as possible to set the stage for a lifelong connection.

So how did I make the leap to yoga for babies? That also goes back to my family. There were always lots of children around, and my mother sang a beautiful poem to welcome each new baby into the family. She sang about a star leaving the heavens to join us on Earth for a lifetime until it returned to its residence in heaven. As a child, I took my mother's words literally and believed that babies were stars from heaven. Today our scientists have proven my mother correct: we are all made of stardust. Our family believed in one basic assumption: Children are not to be formed into what parents want, but to be guided into becoming who they were always meant to be.

I decided that one of the ways this could be accomplished was by mirroring the actions of my grandfather, who, as an animal trainer, used a method now called "horse whispering." I watched him and wanted to do the same with babies and children. I call this concept "baby whispering."

Whispering, whether to animals or people, is about getting synchronized to the rhythms of another so that you can intuit what they feel and what they need in order to bond with them. Then teaching and learning flow easily. I call this connecting spirit to spirit. *Spirit* comes from the Latin word *spiro,* which means "I breathe." Baby whispering is a poetic term describing the spiritual connection of an adult to a baby. It allows you to know what a baby is feeling by intuition. This results in an enduring connection that allows for a profound understanding and bond between you and your baby.

Since I come from a family where nurturing, caring, sharing, and loving are ever-present, it seemed natural for me to take charge and become a little mother when my mother was seriously incapacitated. The same instincts led me to work as a psychologist in a hospital later on in life. It was obvious that all of the nurturing I had provided for my younger brother and sisters at home had played an important role in who I had become, and I wanted to extend my gift of giving to other children. I relied heavily on those same yoga concepts that had kept me centered through my traumatic experiences in childhood.

I eventually became trained as a psychoanalyst, and all of my subsequent research and clinical interests have involved children in some way. Even though I dealt primarily with adults, I could always picture them as children and see the early seeds of difficulty. Through infant stimulation programs that I developed, I became the only clinician on staff who could successfully relate to the needs of both the youngest of babies and their parents. It is this natural skill of relating and connecting to others that I hope to share with you.

As a psychotherapist and licensed yoga practitioner, I encourage parents to relate better to their children. This principle led to the creation of the Goodson Parker Wellness Center in New York City in 1996, where I teach the Yoga Baby program. The program and this book are the result of my many years of research on infant and child development and parent-child relationships. Everything you read here comes straight from my experience—and from my heart, because that's where my love of life, children, and babies come from. I cannot imagine my world without babies or children.

Being able to help a mother and father welcome their new child and begin to bond is the greatest joy for me. It wasn't until I had a child of my own that I truly discovered what a powerful tool yoga can be in bonding with others. It allowed me to relate to my son on a daily basis and helped me develop a greater understanding of children's needs. Over the years, parents have looked to me to change their children into something they are not. What I do and what this book encourages is to help babies and children grow into the unique individuals they are intended to be.

In addition to providing an enhanced emotional bond with your baby, the Baby Yoga program offers an endless list of health benefits to all the systems in both your body and your baby's. Yoga movements stimulate the epidermal, digestive, lymphatic, cardiovascular, and pulmonary systems; they help cleanse the body of toxins and balance the endocrine and nervous systems. Yoga can help decrease heart rate, blood pressure, oxygen consumption, and metabolic rate, and can lower the concentration of lactic acid in the body, thus reducing anxiety. Yoga can align the vertebrae, strengthen the muscles, increase spinal flexibility, lengthen the ligaments, and reduce chronic anxiety.

The Yoga Baby program presented in this book is the result of all my work with babies and their parents at the Goodson Parker Wellness Center. From these learning experiences, I have devised a series of ten sessions during which I teach moms, dads, and caregivers how to do yoga with their babies. I call this the dance between parent and baby, because the purpose is not to teach you how to teach your baby yoga; rather, it is to teach you and your baby how to relate better by learning yoga together. In each session, you will find several exercises for you and several tailored to your baby. In each succeeding session, more exercises will be added until you have a full program outlined for use every day, if you so choose. I believe this program helps create a secure bond between you and your baby, as well as a deeper level of understanding. With Yoga Baby, you can expect to get to know your baby better than you ever have in the past and to appreciate on a new and profound level the magical star you have brought into the world.

The Yoga Baby Program

Life is filled with rhythms. The planet has rhythms: the ebb and flow of the tides, the seasonal changes as Earth journeys around the Sun, the sequence of night and day as the planet spins on its axis. Your body and your baby's body have rhythms also: the heartbeat, the pulse of the blood flowing through the veins, the breath, the pattern of the brain waves, the pulse of the cerebrospinal fluid surrounding the brain.

When the rhythms of the body pull together, there is a coherent and central pulse that becomes the characteristic and identifiable rhythm of the person, like the purr of a cat. Because rhythm is formed by vibrational patterns, we speak of people as having a particular central vibration. Vibrations are said to oscillate like waves and are described by length and frequency. If two or more people vibrate at the same frequency, they are said to be on the same wavelength or in harmony. They have bonded. Once a parent and a baby bond, a parent can intuit the baby's needs. *Yoga Baby* is about teaching you how to bond with your baby so you can parent intuitively. In this way, you are the expert with your baby; the professionals are then your aids.

In this book, I will teach you eight major ways to bond with your baby—spiritually, physically, emotionally, ego-to-ego, empathetically, expressively, mentally, and by empowerment. Each of these corresponds to a different energy center, or chakra, in the body. Getting synchronized will allow you to create a bond of security and trust with your baby that can last a lifetime.

In my experience with the Yoga Baby program, I have found that all new parents are concerned with how to connect with their babies and are somewhat anxious about being physical with them. A tiny newborn, in all his vulnerability, can evoke all of a parent's hopes, dreams, and fears. Yet the establishment of trust and security in the bond between parent and baby can change the baby's life. The Yoga Baby program uses yoga as the medium through which this bond is established. Through Yoga Baby, moms, dads, and other caregivers can learn to be comfortable with and relax around their babies. This sense of security and peace of mind can be transmitted to their infants in our ten-session program, strengthening the parent-baby bond and encouraging greater harmony, ease, security, and even serenity.

Specifically, the Yoga Baby program combines yoga and psychology. The yoga portion of the program is based on hatha yoga, a form that focuses on spinal alignment, and the development of bodily flexibility and strength. It benefits the nervous system, the endocrine system, and the brain, resulting in increased mental focus, greater emotional stability, and an enhanced sense of well-being for both parent and baby.

The Yoga Baby program ties infant development stages to eight energetic centers of the body, which are related to the baby's endocrine and hormonal systems. Specific movements are given to stimulate each of the energetic centers for both baby and parent. I call this "relationship yoga" because parent and baby engage in yoga movements together. As the baby develops, I highlight the developmental task involved in each of these energetic centers and address potential imbalances and difficulties.

These are the seven energetic centers in the human body plus one unofficial addition:

1. **The permanent center** is not an official center, but a location I added. It is situated at the navel, where the umbilical cord is connected, and is psychologically related to being centered and spiritually synchronized.

2. **The root center** is at the coccygeal plexus, is associated with the eliminative organs, and is psychologically related to self-preservation and being physically synchronized.

3. **The regenerative center** is located at the sacral plexus, is associated with the assimilative and sexual organs and glands, and is psychologically related to self-gratification and being synchronized emotionally.

4. **The solar plexus center** is associated with the digestive organs and adrenal glands, and is psychologically related to self-identity and synchronization of the will.

5. **The heart center,** associated with the heart, lungs, and thymus gland, is psychologically related to self-acceptance and being synchronized empathetically.

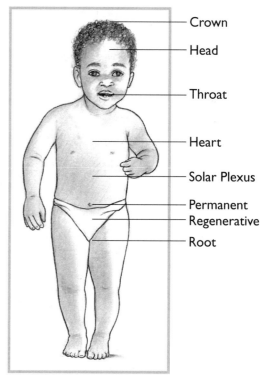

Crown

Head

Throat

Heart

Solar Plexus

Permanent
Regenerative

Root

6. **The throat center** is associated with the thyroid and parathyroid glands and is psychologically related to self-expression and being synchronized expressively.

7. **The head center,** associated with the brain and pituitary gland, is psychologically related to self-reflection and being synchronized mentally.

8. **The crown center,** associated with the pineal gland, is psychologically related to universal identity and being synchronized spiritually.

In the Yoga Baby program, a series of three or four movements is performed several times in order to stimulate different areas of the body. The total number of movements per session may vary from twenty to thirty, depending upon the age of the baby. The point is not the precision of movement but the quality of the relationship as the parent and baby engage in this shared activity.

Psychologists have found that the art of soothing oneself is the most important of psychic tools and that it is learned through a baby's primary relationship to a caregiver. The parent's ability to soothe leaves a child less vulnerable to the vicissitudes of life. We know that emotional learning is critical to brain development, and that the brain develops to two-thirds of its full size during the first three or four years of life. Therefore, what we adults do with our babies, both in utero and after delivery, is of the utmost importance. The Yoga Baby program was developed to amplify emotional learning for you and your baby. Because emotional learning is a lifelong process, it is set in motion with the first and most important relationship, the one between parent and child. This relationship sets the stage for later peer relationships so critical to healthy human development.

You are now ready to embark on what could be the most rewarding experience of your life—bonding with your child. You and your baby will be giving to and receiving from each other your entire lives, a process that started in utero where your baby's connection to you and those close to you existed for nine months, only to continue naturally after the baby is born.

The Yoga Way

Developed in India more than five thousand years ago, yoga is a discipline used to maintain physical and psychological well-being. The benefits of hatha yoga, the form of yogic practice I use in the Yoga Baby program, include improved physical strength and flexibility, mental clarity, greater self-understanding, better stress control, and general well-being. The word *yoga* means "union" in Sanskrit, and the word *hatha* is derived from the two Sanskrit words *ha* and *tha,* meaning "sun" and "moon." Hence hatha yoga is yoga of the Sun and Moon. According to yogic teaching, our bodies are miniature replicas of the solar system. The Sun represents yang, or dynamic, radiant energy, and the Moon represents yin, or magnetic energy; the two together create wholeness or unity. Because the goal of hatha yoga is to bring oneself into harmony with "The Source," one's mental, emotional, and physical faculties—the inner solar system—must be brought into harmony with the external solar system. Inner harmony consists of the alignment of one's physical, emotional, mental, and spiritual faculties with the outer harmony of the Earth and other planets aligned in this galaxy within the universe. Because our babies can be considered miniature replicas of the solar system, in Yoga Baby we sometimes call them our little stars.

The focus of each of our yoga sessions will be on a specific energy center of the body and will consist of movements associated with stimulating that area. An energy center, or chakra, is defined as a vortex of the body that both receives and sends energy. These energy centers coordinate with the physical endocrine system and the hormonal system associated with psychological states. The chakras are considered the points where spirit meets matter and through which vital life energy flows. Yoga is a method of stimulating these centers, which in turn affect both the body and mind. Although these energy centers are said to have a general body location and are described in association with the endocrine system's hormones, they do not actually exist in physical form.

The heart center is said to divide the lower three chakras, which are considered more connected to the Earth and material concerns, from the higher three energy centers, which are more connected to the heavens and spiritual concerns. But I prefer to think of the heart center as unifying the lower three with the higher three. In the Yoga Baby program, movements are designed to progress up the vertical core of the spine from lower to higher. This can be described as ascending from the physical to the spiritual. Yoga focuses on the concept of polarity to obtain not just balance within the person but also balance of the person with the outside world. Energy that flows downward along the spine is considered more related to the physical, and energy that flows upward is more related to the spiritual. In yoga, it is essential to combine the flows of energy both upward and downward to attain balance and create a sense of wholeness.

The development of the energy of the body is such that your baby starts life in utero rolled up in a ball, called the fetal position. It is such a comforting position that even adults will regress to this position in times of stress. From the ball position, the baby is then pushed out head first, but without the physical strength to sit or stand erect. At birth, there are only two curves in the spine, the thoracic and the sacral. The sacral curve includes the five fused bones of the lowest portion of the spine, necessary for the movement of the lower extremities and for the use of the feet in preparation for standing erect. The thoracic curve is the backward curve of the spine in the chest area, necessary for the execution of arm movements and involved in crawling. The energy centers of the body activate over the first year or so, beginning at the very base of the spinal column and gradually working up the vertical core through the backbone as the baby develops. Some call this the tree of life, with the body and its attachments swinging about the trunk of the symbolic tree, the spinal column of the child. From the time the baby develops the ability to hold his head up and make other head movements, the cervical curve, the forward curve of the spine from the inside of the head to the beginning of the neck, develops. As the baby begins to walk, the lumbar curve, the forward curve of the spine in the middle portion of the body, appears, to help with the mobility of the upper and lower extremities. These four curves form the familiar S-curve of the spine.

So the human tree of life develops as the energetic centers activate, stacking up along the spine from sacral to lumbar, to thoracic to cervical curves. Then the structure of the child has all the necessary bends to create an erect body with mobility of movement and stability of structure planted solidly on Earth, yet reaching up to the heavens. Think of the spine as the tree of life, with all the other parts of the body branching off the main trunk. All of this development is based on energy flow.

The Benefits of Yoga

The health benefits of yoga are many: decreases in heart rate, blood pressure, oxygen consumption, metabolic rate, and concentration of lactic acid in the blood; increases in alpha brain wave activity, the brain's resting state for recharging; reduction of anxiety; and deepened relaxation. Some have reported sharpened alertness, increased energy and productivity, increased objectivity and accessibility of emotions, decreased self-criticism, and decreased dependence upon substances such as alcohol and recreational drugs. Many report heightened self-esteem and a stronger self-identity.

Yoga teaches that all life is one and that all living matter is connected. It develops the body as well as the mental and emotional faculties. The type of exercise that Westerners may be accustomed to, such as running and other aerobic activities, emphasizes jerky muscle movements with many repetitions and extreme physical exertion. This produces excessive lactic acid in the muscles, which causes fatigue. In yoga, however, health is considered a state in which all the organs function in harmony under the control of the mind. All movements are slow and gradual, with proper breathing and relaxation.

The main purpose of exercise is to increase circulation and the intake of oxygen. This can be achieved through simple movements of the spine and joints combined with deep breathing. Yogic exercise helps increase the circulation and keeps the arteries elastic through movements that maintain an even supply of blood to every part of the body. If the blood flows steadily and evenly, the body may remain pliable throughout life. Good posture and balance are thought essential to long, elastic ligaments. In yoga, much attention is paid to body alignment and mobility of the spine.

Yogic exercise also focuses on the endocrine glands, which affect the emotions. Yogic postures strengthen the endocrine system and help bring the emotions under control through deep concentration and relaxation. Yoga has been found to counteract the effects of nervous disorders and heart problems.

The Yoga Baby Philosophy

Your baby is a unique person brought into your life for a purpose. The pairing of you with this baby is sheer perfection, no matter the difficulties that may emerge. A perfect match does not mean a lifetime guarantee of no frustration and no problems. Conception occurred with the agreement of mother, father, and baby. The baby creates herself for nine months in utero, where the connection to you existed according to some higher plan for the benefit of both of you. The baby exists in several dimensions and is continually developing physically, emotionally, mentally, and spiritually. But newly born babies are mostly spirit clothed with bodies.

The benefits of the Yoga Baby program include special relating time; more trust and confidence between parent and baby; parental confidence; increased immunity; better sleep, digestion and circulation; neuromuscular development and preparation for the baby's mobility; and better-regulated emotions. This program will help you increase your powers of concentration and patience, aiding you in the task of helping your baby blossom into the person she was always meant to be.

You can use the knowledge of your baby's specific birth circumstances to enhance the benefits of the Yoga Baby program. For example, the circumstances of birth may be related to later personality issues, not merely developmental issues. Take note of such questions as:

1. *Was the baby born in a breech presentation?* Observe whether the baby is slow to make the transition from one activity to another or from one person to another. Is the child slow to leave one place and reluctant to enter another? Is the child resistant to being pushed or insistent on doing things her own way in her own time? In the Yoga Baby program, allow your baby extra transition time.

2. *Was the birth fast?* Look for eagerness, impatience to get on with matters, and sometimes impulsiveness (a tendency to leap before looking). In the program, allow for more movements and shorter sequences of each movement.

3. *Was the birth induced?* Look for stubbornness and a tendency to just stop in the middle of activities. Some of the most obstinate children have had an induced birth. In the program, allow the baby to stop,

and then resume the movements slowly and gradually. Work with, not against, the baby's resistance and at the baby's pace.

There are exceptions to all these examples, but it is clear to me that circumstances of birth do indicate something about emerging personality and the need to make modifications in the program.

Especially for Fathers

You can become as adept as your wife in caring for your baby. You do not have to abdicate totally to Mom during baby-bonding time. You have an important place in this process also. Yoga Baby is an excellent way to get involved with your newborn. The program can help bring you a feeling of empowerment and begin the bonding between you and your baby as early as possible.

Fathers sometimes feel left out by Mom's constant attention to baby. If you and your wife have had a particularly intense and loving relationship, you may feel as if you have lost your partner because of her preoccupation with the baby and/or shut out of the baby's life as well. This is especially so during the first six weeks of the newborn's life. If it is possible for you to be patient during these initial stages of a mother's love affair with her new baby, I would suggest that this is the best route for getting right back to the top of the list. If your uneasiness creates conflict for the mother, she may find her role as mother even more difficult and may focus more attention on the child. Find ways to participate with your mate in caring for the baby. There may be practical rewards as well; for example, you may be the one who develops the magic touch for alleviating colic.

Become as competent as your wife at caring for the baby so that she feels more and more relaxed about loosening her tight grip. If you can allow the process to unfold, your mate will be rejuvenated in her interest and focus on you, and will involve you in more activities with the baby in the very near future.

Especially for Caregivers

Babies need more than feeding and diapering. Even though the baby you care for is not your own, remember that all babies need love and that your attitude toward this baby is conveyed all the time, not only at every feeding and diapering event. Try to clear your own personal issues to provide for the needs of this baby, which has been delivered to your care as a gift to you. If you are caring for this baby as part of your job, loving this baby does not take away love from your own children. Love is an ever-expanding phenomenon; the more love you make, the more there is to make, so give yourself permission to love your own children and to love this baby as well. You are a valued and important part of this child's life, and what you do now will have an impact on this baby for a long time.

It is essential to allow as much physical play as this baby wants. Sometimes caregivers are so conscientious about doing a proper job that they are especially protective of a baby and may inadvertently restrain the baby too much in the interests of keeping him safe. Try to be sure to allow for safe yet free physical exploration for the baby. It is essential for his brain development.

Special-needs Babies

Sara was a special-needs child with a slight case of cerebral palsy, though her mother came into the class without any particular mention of Sara's needs. I realized very quickly that Sara was delayed in her development and not able to control her body as well as the other babies. Sara's mother held back whenever the positions and movements were demonstrated and the other mothers were imitating the movements. As she sat quietly, she clutched her daughter. She was obviously protecting Sara from the others' gazes and from my possible judgment that something was wrong.

First I began to work on releasing some of the mother's tension in her back, which required that she put Sara down on the blanket for a moment. As we proceeded, it was clear that the mother wanted Sara to receive all the positive benefits available to any other child. I worked gently with little Sara's tummy. Over the course of the session, Sara's mom began to release some of her own body tension and fear, and then Sara began to relax and have a good time. It was essential for Sara's mom to feel Sara was accepted and not judged. Since one of my passions is working with special-needs babies, this was an easy assignment. Sara continued with us, and just like any other baby, she had a good time and enjoyed bonding with her mother. Plus her mom has learned some wonderful strategies for working with her daughter.

Special-needs children, including those with birth complications and/or mental, physical, or emotional delays—assuming they have clearance from their pediatrician—benefit equally from the Yoga Baby program, with certain modifications.

Multiple Births

When you are caring for the survival needs of more than one baby, you may feel pulled in so many directions that you fear losing your own centeredness. It is essential that you stay as centered as you can; if certain negative feelings come up, such as anger or frustration, find a place or a way to express them and then move on. Do not be afraid to ask others for help when you need it. Everyone has a limit to their abilities, and when you feel close to your limit, seek help.

Adopted Babies

It's important for adoptive mothers to understand that their babies *do* have a connection to them. If a baby was nurtured for nine months by a biological mother and then adopted by another, I believe there's still a match; it was no accident that this particular family received this particular child. Therefore, think of your adopted baby as a magical gift to your adoptive family, no matter the circumstances of adoption.

Adoptive mothers should realize that it's never too late to bond with the baby and to feel as if she had really been inside your body. Focus on connecting to the rhythms of your baby even though the baby is no longer in utero. Pay particular attention to the directions in the following exercises for sensing the baby's rhythms.

One client of mine who has an adopted son seemed very hesitant and a bit jealous of the moms who had actually borne their children— she presumed they found mothering more natural, and therefore easier. She was struggling with the mothering process, was very unsure of herself, and seemed anxious about forging a bond with her baby. As the first session proceeded, she was able to see that the other mothers did not have nearly as much of an advantage as she had thought. She had an instinctive touch for her son, Sam, and as her confidence increased, he responded; it was clear he had been hesitant with her precisely because she was tenuous with him. When some of the other mothers asked her for pointers on her magic touch, she was clearly delighted. She possessed maternal skills she had not even realized—her fear had blocked their expression. By the end of the session, she was thrilled with herself and little Sam and she clearly felt empowered. Although one session does not cure a long-term problem, this adoptive mother had gained a new perspective.

Note: At the end of each chapter, when applicable, I will include pertinent information and/or tips for fathers, caregivers, special-needs babies, multiple births, and adopted babies under the appropriate heading.

Getting Started

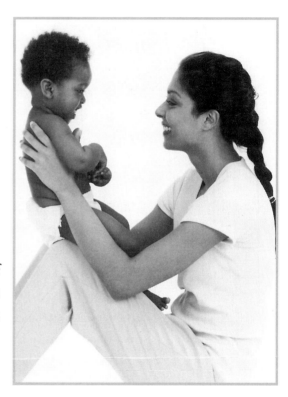

Now that you've had a preview of yoga and how it can strengthen the bonds between you and your baby, here's what you need to know to prepare for your first session.

A Safe Place

Choose a location that's dimly lit, quiet, and soothing. Don't place yourself in direct sunlight, since babies are sensitive to light. Look for a room in your home that's quiet and clean with minimal furniture and few visual distractions. A carpeted floor or a padded mat with cushioning is preferred. It's best to use the same room or even the same portion of a room each time so that the baby starts to associate the space with time for connecting with you.

Clean Up Your Act

Keep the area where you hold your yoga session clean. If the baby spits up or spoils the area, it should be cleaned immediately so that the baby gets accustomed to working in a very hygienic environment. Yoga is about cleansing and purifying oneself, and the environment should reinforce this ideal.

Practicing a Ritual

Many people enjoy adding a ritual component to their Yoga Baby sessions. Ritual is a way to make the ordinary experiences of life extraordinary. It is a way to connect our day-to-day lives to the spiritual world. It brings greater meaning to our sense of purpose. Therefore, I am in favor of adding ritual to your sessions—in the form of music or flowers, for instance—to enhance your enjoyment of the Yoga Baby program. Because Yoga Baby is an experience, ritual is one way to heighten that experience. It is an aid in helping parent and baby on all levels: physically, emotionally, mentally, and spiritually.

You might link each session with a milestone in your newborn's life. We celebrate each energetic center by focusing on the unique quality of each in the development of a baby. Here is the schedule I like to follow but feel free to modify this to suit yourself:

- When your baby *arrives home from the hospital,* celebrate the permanent center and the mystery of conception and delivery.

- At the *two-week birthday,* celebrate the root center and the baby's will to live.
- After *one month,* celebrate the regenerative center for the delight of being here to enjoy the Earth.
- At *two months,* celebrate the solar plexus and the emerging personality of the baby.
- When she reaches *three months,* celebrate the heart center and the love you share.
- At *four months* old, celebrate the throat center and all the sounds the baby makes.
- At the *five-month birthday,* celebrate the head center and the developing mental abilities of the brain and eyes.
- Celebrate the crown center and the baby's connection to the universe at the *six-month birthday.*

In each of the following sections, you'll find suggestions regarding the inclusion of certain scents, colors, and sounds to add to the enjoyment of rituals you can perform for that particular chakra. These are merely rough guides. Proceed with the Yoga Baby program as you wish, but create your rituals as a meaningful way to amplify the experience of each energetic center as you bond with your baby. Each of the energetic centers has its own unique quality that allows you to connect to your baby in a particular way. Some people try to define a center by a particular color or specific sound for the chakra; I usually find this too confining and rigid. I prefer to create a mood that adds to the yoga experience.

I start by using colors that have a personal meaning for me and remind me of the center. The colors I choose may change over time. Then I select background music that I associate with the center, and I modify the lighting to create a restful mood. I burn incense before the session (never when the baby is present) to clear the air, selecting a scent that has some association with the center being addressed. Be sure to avoid heavy scents that may irritate the baby; try sage, which is light. If there are fresh flowers available, I try to have those that remind me of the center placed around the room. I place mats on the floor, provide extra pillows for bracing backs, and have cloth diapers available in case of soiling. I always begin each session by washing my hands with antibacterial soap, removing all jewelry, and applying lotion to my hands to be sure they are soft.

Time After Time

Try to do the activity each day at the same time. The afternoon is prime time for yoga, because the baby's body is fully warmed up and fed and there is nothing to keep her from truly focusing. But if you get home from the office at 7 P.M. and feel this would be a good time for a yoga session, that's fine, too.

If you don't think you have time during your hectic day, try this time-management exercise: write down what you do all day, and you will most likely discover some free time where you can easily fit in a brief yoga session. If you can pinpoint a few free moments throughout your day, try to arrange your schedule so that they are lumped together to give you a solid time slot for your yoga practice. Keep the first sessions short, about ten minutes each, and gradually lengthen the time for a session to approximately twenty to thirty minutes.

Food for Thought

Throughout the day, eat small, light, easily digestible meals that are high in complex carbohydrates and low in fat. Low-sugar cereals, salads, fresh fruit, vegetables, whole-grain breads and pastas, and brown rice are good options; heavier foods, such as those with cream sauces and butter, should be avoided. If you still need an energy boost, try a glass of juice or a cup of soup about an hour before class. Most yoga practitioners are vegetarian because a diet containing much meat is not conducive to yogic practice. Avoid feeding your baby for one and a half to two hours prior to the session. If necessary during a session, of course, your baby may have water or even a little milk. But it is best if all these physical needs are taken care of beforehand. You should avoid eating at least one hour before starting your yoga session. Nursing moms need lots of liquids, though, so keep water on hand.

Dress Code

You can do yoga in any comfortable clothing. Go for exercise gear for maximum freedom of movement. A diaper or no clothing at all is best for the baby as long as she is kept warm. If your baby is naked, be sure your exercise pad is water-resistant, because your baby may soil it.

Baby's Actions Speak Louder Than Words

To get you and your baby into yoga mode, observe your baby and become familiar with her physical characteristics and facial and body movements. Your baby can't tell you what she is feeling, so you need to observe her carefully.

Look at her to try to get a sense of how she moves her body. Some babies furl up as if they are still in utero, where the water environment of amniotic fluid leads to the baby's compressed body. You need to lengthen the baby gently to prepare her for her earthly existence in this air environment, where the baby's body can expand and where an unfurled body is necessary. Notice if she curls one foot in a particular direction or moves both feet. How does she move her hands? Are they all scrunched up? Does she keep her hands curled up close to the body? Will she let you gently coerce them away from the body? Will she let you open the hand and then the fingers? Or does she resist? Will she let you lengthen the legs? Or does she resist? Wherever you encounter resistance, do not force the movement.

In these ten sessions, you will gradually help your baby release and lengthen. At this point, you should be observing and making notes for work in future sessions. Note which side of the body, right or left, she seems more able to move freely. If there is a favoring of one side or the other, encourage the baby to move on the other side, for balance. If she turns her head mostly to the left, urge her also to turn it to the right. Make notations of how the baby uses her body and its energy flow. Look deeply into those new eyes and try to get a sense of the person who is housed inside. Try to get a sense of her temperament and personality. This is the beginning of learning who your baby is.

Get into Position

Yoga technique involves the use of polarities—as one example, while you're gently moving the baby's muscles in one direction with one hand, your other hand is moving the opposing muscles in the opposite direction with equal, gentle force.

The technique, or rather art, of yoga is more important than the actual physical movement and postures, because all movements are done reaching deeply into the earth while ascending in equal effort toward the heavens. This allows the entire body to stretch gradually, leading to overall good health. You will be moving your baby in these directions because your baby needs your help, but always work gently. I urge you to try all movements on a rag doll first, before working on your baby. Yoga constantly moves toward balanced body use. If the baby has a tendency to flex certain muscles, for example, yoga encourages extension of those muscles so that the baby begins to get some sense of balance in body use.

The Right Frame of Mind

Clear your mind of any troubles and emotional upset at the start of each session, because these will affect the baby. Moms can relax through a series of deep-breathing exercises like this one: Breathe in through the nose for five counts, hold for two counts, then breathe out through the nose for five counts and repeat for several minutes. Through this inhale-exhale pattern, focus on breathing more and more deeply into the belly. This will help empty your mind of all the troubles of the day—at least for the duration of the session. Your baby may begin a session in any number of emotional states but will usually leave the session in a very relaxed and contented mood.

Holding Baby

Place your baby on his back by holding the back of the head with one hand and supporting the lower back with the other hand. Gently put your baby down on the pad and remove your hands from underneath. Never let the neck be overstressed.

If Baby Is Sick

Skip your yoga session if your baby is sick. However, yoga can sometimes settle a mild case of colic.

How to Proceed with the Yoga Baby Program

The chapters in this book are arranged so that you and your baby will be working your way through the Yoga Baby program. Start with the first session and try one or two sessions a week, but don't do more than one session's worth of exercises in one sitting. Notice how your baby reacts to these new movements in order to determine how to proceed. You may increase the frequency of the sessions or the length of each if your baby is enjoying them. Once you have gone through the complete ten sessions in order and are familiar with the program in its entirety, feel free to change the order of the exercises and make other modifications that suit you.

I recommend that parents do yoga at least two or three times per week, although I think it is wonderful if you can do it every day. I did yoga every day with my son and found that it became our special relating time. Throughout his life, we always found an hour a day to relate through yoga; during these sessions, no interruptions from the outside world were allowed. I have seen the tremendous difference this special time made in his development.

Postures for Moms and Babies

Each chapter will describe different postures for both you and your baby to try. First try the movement yourself so that you are in a comfortable position to then work with your baby. This should also capture the baby's attention. She will be mesmerized by what you are doing.

Adapting the Yoga Baby Program for Your Baby's Age Group

Each chapter in the book will target two main age groups: from birth to six months, and from six to twelve months. A follow-up chapter will address the needs of babies from twelve to twenty-four months, as well as ways to keep you and your child active in the practice of yoga as she gets older.

Dos and Don'ts

Here are some basic dos and don'ts that will help you prepare for the Yoga Baby program. Follow them to establish a sound bond between you and your baby.

DO . . .

- Tune in to your baby's body language. Your baby will let you know what she likes or dislikes. Match your hand pressure and movements to your baby's preference. Some like firm pressure, while others prefer a softer touch; some prefer the feel of a moving hand, and other babies respond better to a still hand.
- Talk softly, lowering your voice to a gentle whisper. Even a newborn knows your voice, from the time he spent in utero, and finds it comforting. Adopted babies are still getting to know your voice; use it softly and reassuringly.
- Use a gentle touch on the baby's skin.
- Hold your baby firmly and reassuringly.

- Be kind to your body and slow down all your movements. Try moving slowly, and then slow down even more. If you push too hard as you are performing a movement, you may feel uncomfortable and you will not enjoy it.
- Focus totally on your baby for the entire session.

DON'T . . .

- Violate your baby's personal space. Do not work any closer to your baby than your baby is comfortable with.
- Make loud noises around your baby.
- Talk on the telephone or answer the doorbell during a session.
- Overstimulate your baby by doing too many things at once during a session.
- Continue when baby has become tired. There's always tomorrow.
- Have visitors observing the session until you have developed your skills and both you and the baby are comfortable with the movements.

Getting Started: Commonly Asked Questions

Q: How do I know if I'm doing it right?

A: For yourself, you will experience an exhilarating feeling of opening and release. If you do not feel this, you have probably not made all the body adjustments necessary to provide that full opening feeling. Some of the poses may be uncomfortable at first. Gently coax yourself into them and continue holding according to the directions. In your baby, you will notice the emotional reactions. At first your child may react negatively to these new exercises, but once she adjusts, she should begin accepting the stimulation pleasantly. Most babies are tired at the end of the sessions and may get a little fussy before falling asleep.

Q: Is it okay to do yoga to music?

A: If you warm up with movements that open up your hips and shoulders, why not open up your ears as well? It's a matter of personal preference, but you should skip music that's distracting or not conducive to relaxation, such as heavy metal, grunge, or rap. Instead, opt for soothing chamber pieces, tapes of natural ocean sounds, or New Age music that induces a meditative state. Many babies like the soothing sounds.

Q: How do I know when I'm ready to graduate to the next level?

A: Your goal is to always feel focused and yet to achieve an altered state. I have given variations for some poses, but every pose has both gentler and more demanding variations, and you can adopt a pose to your needs at any level. You should shift your pose to an easier position if you start to feel physically stressed, but remember that even the simplest of poses still benefits advanced practitioners, because the mind is always engaged.

The Permanent Center

BONDING SPIRITUALLY

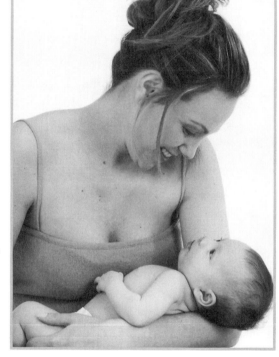

Antonia tended to have mild colic on a regular basis, and I realized at the start of our Yoga Baby sessions that she was uncomfortable. I discovered that if I placed Antonia over my knees so that she could bend backward with support, and then massaged her very gently in the manner described in this chapter (see Belly Cupping exercise, page 44), it would alleviate a great deal, if not all, of the colic. Then we could begin a regular session. The initial work of relieving her distress seemed to be the ideal method for her to proceed.

In order to forge a union between you and your baby and establish a mutual connection, we will begin with the center of the baby's body, the belly, which I call the permanent center. Work with this center to bond spiritually with your baby, accentuating the importance of welcoming this unique star to our Earth.

The permanent center may be described metaphorically as the originating spark for the artistic creation that we call life. The permanent center is the originating point in consciousness of your baby's entire existence and the point from which he creates himself in the womb. Consider conception as your baby's own version of the big bang, where his life originates and from which point it continues to unfold. Your baby's permanent center is activated between conception and birth. For nine months, his entire connection to you was through the umbilical cord—your body met all of his needs for nurturing, assimilation, and elimination. Via the blood you shared, received information, including tastes and emotions, was filtered through you. The umbilicus is your child's first connection to something outside himself. From the start we are all connected to someone else. All people have a belly button as a lifelong memento of this connection.

This center of gravity is a position where great comfort can occur and where the baby will later pull all his levels of self together to feel "centered." The key word for this center is "ongoing," because it indicates the ongoing nature of consciousness from this originating point. The navel truly represents your baby's most important connection to you—even after the umbilical cord is no longer attached. Some call this permanent connection the silver chord, indicating an ongoing connection to the stars and to the Earth. After the cord is cut, your baby may no longer receive physical nourishment from you internally, but you continue to nourish him externally and emotionally. Symbolically, the cord is cut so the relationship between mother and baby may shift from physical union in the womb to an emotional attachment outside the womb, as you are now two separate beings capable of developing a bond. Because of the great significance of this permanent center, a baby receives much comfort from stimulation in the area around the navel.

Whenever I think of this center, in the middle of the tummy, I am reminded of my son at age three looking down and examining his navel. He had just started watching *Sesame Street* and he asked, "Who put the *O* in my tummy?" I suppose he was in the earliest stages of what is often called "contemplating one's navel"—which really means examining one's origins.

When the umbilical cord is cut, the invisible chord between baby and mom does not really disappear—it continues invisibly for a lifetime. The more in harmony you two are, the easier your child's ongoing development will be. Therefore, I focus on methods for moms to synchronize themselves to their baby through the baby's own rhythms, such as heartbeat, breath, and pulse of the cerebrospinal fluid. In every way, I try to help moms sense these rhythms and match their own rhythm to their baby's.

Physical Purpose

This session focuses on stimulating your baby's permanent center, providing comfort and security for his basic needs. This central part of your baby is his center of gravity, and it provides the center of his physical power to help him operate and execute the physical movements and exercises needed for his entire life.

Psychological Purpose

Psychologically, we feel centered when all levels of self—physical, emotional, mental, and spiritual—are pulled together and working toward a clear goal. When this isn't so, we feel split, divided, fragmented. The aim of this session is to provide a feeling of being centered. After the baby leaves the watery womb to enter the outside world, this center allows him to trust that he is still safe and will still have his basic needs met. The first few months are about survival and the child's developing awareness that he is all right and is being cared for. Babies love to be comforted and patted right there on the tummy. An open permanent center brings with it a clear sense of feeling centered and belonging. Whenever there is a closed center, it brings alienation from others and a sense of being adrift. We call such people "lost souls."

Babies whose basic needs routinely are not met early in their development develop enormous fear and tightness in the midsection, leading to all sorts of digestive, assimilative, and eliminative difficulties. Therefore, your attention to your baby's most basic needs in the first few months of life should be vigilantly guarded. He relies on you to anticipate his most basic needs because he cannot yet do much of anything for himself. He needs you in the most basic of ways—to survive.

Yoga Mind

The permanent center is the mini–Big Bang for your baby, where he began his consciousness in this life. It is the beginning, the origin, of his universe.

Yoga Technique

Consciousness exists on many levels at all times, no matter how young the baby—even when in the womb. Therefore, yoga technique is careful with all external and internal stimulation that a baby is exposed to, whether before or after birth. The conversation and emotional tone a mother exposes her baby to before birth is as important as the foods the mother eats that affect the growth of the baby.

Ritual

For the permanent center, the scent for centering and relieving anxiety might be sandalwood. The colors might include silver, for the silver chord of life. The music can be any repetitive, hypnotic sounds, so that there seems to be no beginning, no middle, and no ending. Some people think music by Philip Glass exemplifies this. It should have a circular, unending quality, to signify the ongoing nature of consciousness.

The Setup

Once you've found a comfortable position, you should allow about ten minutes to go through the first session with your baby. Sit with your back against a wall or a firm pillow. Unless specified otherwise, most of the movements in this book can be done in one of two positions: with your legs straight out in front of you in an open-legged V position, stretching your inner thighs and extending your back, or in a half-lotus position (similar to sitting cross-legged but with one ankle resting on top of the opposite knee). The baby will usually be placed faceup on the floor on a padded blanket between your legs, or in front of your crossed legs with his head farthest away from your body so he can easily see you at all times. This creates a circle of energy, warmth, and security for the baby as the work begins, and it allows you to readily lift and cuddle your baby at any time for reassurance. As you assume different yoga positions, stay close to your baby so that he feels constantly involved. There is no rigid posture in this work. The technique and process are what count. Remember that all other postures require a strong center and the use of the abdominal muscles so that the center can become the basis for all future movement and exercise. The exercises for the permanent center are the same for all ages from birth to twelve months.

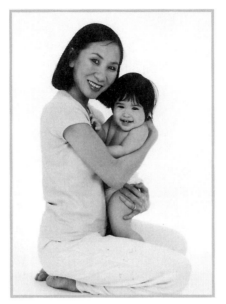

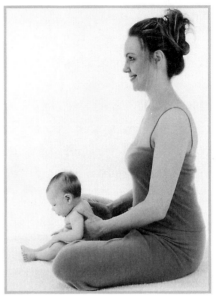

POSTURES FOR MOM   POSTURES FOR MOM

Postures for Mom

By now, you should have discovered a basic position that you feel comfortable in, one that allows you to focus on your baby and lets him focus on you. If you did the first few moves in a cross-legged position, try switching to the V position or kneeling then sitting back on your heels with your feet tucked under your buttocks, so you have more height over your baby and can get a better overview of his reactions to your movements.

BELLY BREATHING

1. With your baby lying on the floor in front of you, begin to focus on your own belly. Breathe deeply into your belly so that the breaths are taken into the spots where you may still be sore from delivery.

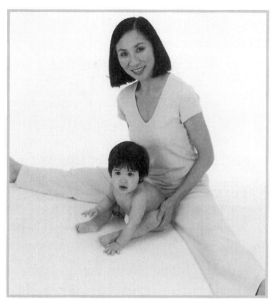

POSTURES FOR MOM

2. Start with deep breathing in slow counts so that your breath goes deep and wide through your front and back. Do this for five repetitions, inhaling and exhaling for the same number of counts, or until the baby gets restless, in which case you should pick her up and comfort her while still breathing deeply. This usually calms the baby, and your breath will begin to be in rhythm with the baby's.

BELLY RUBBING

1. With one hand on your baby's stomach, rub your own belly slowly in circles with the other hand. You may use either hand. Use your whole hand so that you feel the warmth of your hand against your belly. This is very comforting for stomach distress.

2. The strokes should be circular in a clockwise direction, and gentle, never hard or forced. Pregnant mothers do this naturally, but once they deliver the baby they often forget the comfort of this process.

There is no need to hold your stomach in; just let it do whatever feels comfortable. Do this for at least thirty slow strokes, or for three to five minutes.

COLON TRACING

1. With your hand still on your baby's stomach, use your fingertips to trace your colon in a continuous ascending motion up the right side of your body—from the bottom of the inside of the hipbone to the top of the inside of the hipbone.
2. Next, move your hand across your stomach from the right to the left along the transverse colon.
3. Then descend the colon down the left side of your body—from the top of the inside of the hipbone to the bottom of the inside of the hipbone, tracing these parts with your fingers on the outside of the belly. This will allow you to become familiar with your colon area and permanent center so that you will recognize them on your baby in future movements.
4. Repeat five times.

PELVIC RAISES

1. If you are in a kneeling or cross-legged position, switch to a V position. The baby should have a comfortable view of your face and be lying on the floor in front of you.
2. Raise your legs in their V position to encourage a gentle pelvic-floor lift.
3. Drop your legs to feel the lift and release of the lower pelvis. This is a part of the body that is often exhausted from pregnancy and delivery.
4. Repeat five times.

Postures for Baby

From tummy rubbing to basic breathing, you are about to create a very special bond with your baby. Follow these postures in the order in which they are listed here and concentrate on feeling the connection between yourself and your baby. Note that the younger your baby, the shorter the session should be. Sometimes as little as three to five minutes will be enough to begin. Check to be sure he is not hungry and has not soiled himself before proceeding to the next exercise in the session. You can always stop and rest a bit, then begin again.

SENSE THE RHYTHM

1. Place your preferred hand (right hand for right-handed people and left hand for left-handed people) gently on your baby's stomach and feel the rhythms of her breath and her stomach gurgling. Differentiate the two rhythms; how do they sound? You'll feel the expansion and contraction of breath and the lift of the diaphragm, as well as the stomach churning.

2. Now try using your nonpreferred hand (you'll sense different things with different hands); what do you feel? Bond with your baby by joining your breath with hers. Feel her rhythm, then match it.

3. After a few breaths, you will be breathing in unison, which will be very comforting to both you and your baby. The hand is an extension of heart energy, and you can send loving, comforting heart energy through your hands. A calming hand on the baby's belly is a way for her to stay connected and know that she is being held steady by her mom. She can feel comforted, centered, and supported emotionally. Do this for three to five minutes.

COLON TRACING

1. Start by tracing your baby's colon in a gentle, slow massage with the first two fingers of one hand while ascending the colon up the right side of his body.

2. Move to the transverse colon, running across the navel area from the right side to the left.

3. Then move to the descending colon down the left side of the body. This technique will be useful in case your baby develops colic. Babies with colic often pull their legs tighter into their body and seem as if they are in spasm. Don't be afraid to use your hand to smooth the area that seems to be in spasm; the warmth of a hand can be helpful in relieving the distress. Babies respond very well to this. It is also a great way to relieve gas pains.

4. Do this five times.

BELLY BREATHING

1. To encourage belly breathing, which babies often do naturally as
    they inhale, wait till your baby inhales. After she breathes in, cup her
    buttocks and legs together in one hand and bring her legs up to her
    stomach, bending the knees, for just a few moments. Hold this posi-
    tion while the baby inhales and exhales several times.
2. Then release the legs as the baby exhales. This simple movement
    encourages deeper breathing. Do this five times, always in conjunc-
    tion with your baby's breath.

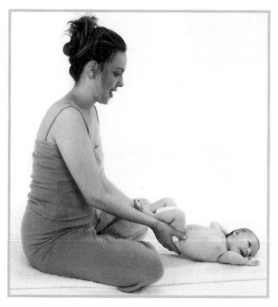

BELLY BREATHING

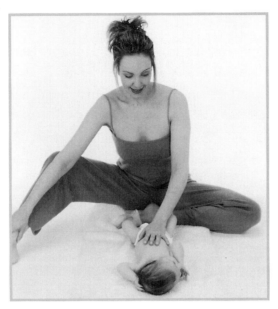

BELLY CUPPING

BELLY CUPPING

This form of touch is designed to provide a gentle massage to the internal organs and exterior skin.

1. Take the baby's whole belly and cup it with one or both hands, depending on how small or large it is. Feel the baby inhale.
2. As the baby is about to release his breath, release the hold gently.
3. Take hold again as the baby is inhaling a breath. The baby's reaction should be contented. Remember that gentle massage of the belly stimulates digestion and encourages the natural release of gas.
4. Do this five times. Rest for a few seconds in between the repetitions.

Observations

Take note of the reactions from your baby throughout the session so you become familiar with what he likes and dislikes. This will help you determine what to expect in future sessions.

Did your baby get quiet through the session or become progressively noisier? If your child became noisy, check your touch; it may not be right for him. Some babies like to be held, some do not. What about your baby?

Does he like to push against something with his feet, arms or body? Pushing is easier than pulling, since he does not yet have the strength to pull.

Commonly Asked Questions

Q: Why do babies need to relax? Aren't they relaxed already?

A: Babies need to adjust from being in a liquid environment to being in an air environment. They also need to learn how to react to their parents, since it's the first time they're dealing with other human beings. They often sense the stress of parents who are not accustomed to taking care of a child. Anxiety can be contagious, even to babies.

Q: I can't get my baby to look at me during a session. What should I do?

A: To get your baby's attention, try speaking to him continuously in a slow, soft voice that will be soothing to his ears. In addition, perform your movements close to him—stretch your back so that your face is near his—so that he feels your presence at all times.

Q: It's difficult for me to let go of the traumas of my day during our yoga session. How can I clear my mind of these obstacles so that I can spend more quality time with my baby?

A: The slow, deep-breathing exercises are key (see Belly Breathing exercise, page 43). Visualize each intrusive thought as a floating leaf drifting down from a tree and accumulating in a pile that you put in a container. Put the container outside the door, to be retrieved at the end of the session. Be easy on yourself when your mind wanders, and bring it gently back to the program.

Multiple Births

If you have been fortunate enough to deliver more than one baby at a time, then you may use Yoga Baby for several babies simultaneously. Many movements can be performed on two babies at the same time. For example, belly cupping can be done with the mother placing one hand on each baby. Take turns by working with one or two babies and letting the other(s) lie flat. The hardest part is deciding whether to focus attention on more than one baby at a time. If you focus on two at the same time, be sure to send energy to each. If you wish to alternate, then focus on one while allowing the other(s) to squirm. Remain as calm and focused as possible.

The Root Center

BONDING PHYSICALLY

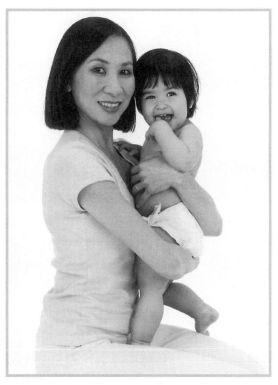

Sally's mom seemed to feel parenting was a battle over who was in charge. So she set about creating a rigid schedule for Sally that included feeding, sleeping, diapering, and activities. This agenda was based on a pediatrician's general recommendations for most babies Sally's age (three months old), but not specifically tailored for Sally. If Sally arrived a little late for class because burping or napping took a little longer, her mother was upset and apologized for her. Sally's mom felt it was a measure of her success as a mother to get Sally on a schedule.

But it takes a bit of time for a baby to settle into a schedule, and that schedule may suddenly shift as the baby develops. While a schedule can help you manage this new part of your life as a parent, you must be flexible; most babies (and children) do not do well with too rigid a schedule.

In working with Sally's root center, I encouraged her mom to spend time with one hand on her own stomach and the other on Sally to sense the differences in the rhythms of their bodies. From week to week, her observations of Sally changed. The child still had not settled into a predictable rhythm, and her bowel movements were not dependably timed. Even extra feedings between scheduled feedings seemed necessary for Sally. As we worked together, her mom began to be more baby-focused and to develop routines that better suited Sally. If Sally tired in the middle of a session, I insisted that they take a break and continue the next day. Although she complained that Sally had not gotten her full session, I suggested the two of them hang out and observe the others. Gradually Sally's mom relaxed and got into the flow of what I call "yoga time," during which the goal is to take things as they come and never force anything. Only then did Sally seem to become more predictably rhythmic.

"The deeper the roots, the higher the tree can grow." That proverb perfectly describes the focus of this session, the root center, through which parents bond physically with their baby. I call this area the baby's generator, since the root center is where life is generated. Every generator needs fuel to generate energy; your baby needs enough fuel to sustain her life and strengthen her will to live. We mothers give birth from this center, and it will be your baby's focus for the first year of life. Although most of the root center's functions are about physical survival, we know that babies who are given adequate food but who are not emotionally nurtured do not thrive. They even run the risk of not surviving. Both physical and emotional nurturing—which you will stimulate in your baby's root center—are necessary to sustain the life of your baby until your baby has enough energy to sustain her own life.

If the permanent center is the originating spark of the artwork that is life, the root center is the generator of all the energy required to accomplish everything your life's work requires. It is the place where all your basic survival needs are met.

Developing most prominently from birth to twelve months, the root center is the energetic center situated at the base of the spinal column. It can be found by locating the perineal muscle, which extends from the tailbone to the pubic bone. The muscle is in the shape of a figure eight, swirling around the anal opening and extending forward to either the vaginal opening for a girl or the scrotum for a boy. Since the ∞ is the symbol for infinity, I call this mark, which is stamped into our human body from the moment of our arrival here on Earth, our "infinite imprint."

A mother who has recently delivered can sense her own root center because it is the pelvic floor that feels so present during menstruation, pregnancy, and delivery. During pregnancy, the pelvic floor gradually lowers with the increasing weight of the developing fetus until during birth most of the root center energy is used to push the new life out into the world.

After delivery of a newborn, this perineal area is tender and sore, particularly if you have had an episiotomy, a surgical procedure for widening the birth opening to facilitate easier delivery. Therefore, all physical stimulation in the perineal area should be done gently. As the baby matures, she will become more mobile, and your healing will coincide with this increased infant activity level; in a few months, you will be able to use these muscles more vigorously. This is necessary for the rigors of caring for an active baby and for sexual reconnection with your mate.

You can sense the pelvic floor—the root center—by practicing the interruption of the flow of urine while sitting on the toilet. When you contract the perineum, the pelvic floor lifts and holds, closing the root center. After birth, the pelvic-floor muscles must regain their tone. This usually occurs gradually, after several months of healing.

The purpose of the movements in this session is to lengthen your baby's legs and feet so that the energy from the root center moves down into the lower extremities, helping to ground her and allowing her to use her legs and ultimately to walk.

The first months of life are related to the physicality of survival, and all of your rapidly growing baby's needs are focused on eating and eliminating. You may notice that your baby exhibits a strong oral focus and tends to turn her mouth and attempt to suckle on whatever stimulates the mouth area. This is called "rooting" behavior; as the root center is connected to the organs of elimination, the bladder and the colon, you can see the link between the intake of nourishment and the elimination of waste as part of the process of becoming rooted to the Earth. When the baby takes in food, she is fueling the generator of the root center. As her sucking and eating urges are satisfied, your baby will learn she can trust the adult world to provide for her needs. Practically speaking, the root center is where your baby's body begins to learn how to process food in an air environment in order to provide for her physical needs. When these needs are adequately met, your baby feels her right to be here, and her will to live is energized.

Physical Purpose

In this session, you will bond physically with your baby and learn how to predict her needs. If you are a nursing mother, you are already physically attuned to your baby because your body becomes anxious to deliver milk at approximately the same time your baby cries out for it. This connection is not limited by physical boundaries, since it can happen whether you are next to your baby or far away. If you are not lactating but using bottles, you may still be physically attuned to your baby. You may sense your baby's emerging hunger before she begins fretting and find yourself preparing a bottle so that it is ready at just the moment your baby begins to cry for milk. Anticipation of your baby's physical needs is an example of bonding physically.

Mere physical sustenance, however, is not enough to help babies grow; they need the love that accompanies sustenance to be fully sustained on Earth. There is no loving gesture greater than warm hands delivering food, so as you feed your baby, check your mood to be sure you are sending love with every drop of milk. When feeding your baby, dismiss your own anger, upset, and resentment, as well as any unnecessary intrusions, so that through the process of nursing, you will be sending both milk and positive feelings to your child.

Psychological Purpose

Through the root center, you will learn to allow and foster your baby's physical growth so that her motor skills and the development of her brain, as well as her sense of exploration, can begin. It is this exploration of the environment and the people around her that allows your baby's brain to develop. In doing so, you are continuing to establish a trusting relationship with your baby. When your baby has a physical need, you provide for it, so she senses that she is being cared for and is wanted and valued. Within the first twelve months, she develops a sense of object permanence, which means that objects that disappear from vision still continue to exist in her mind. This is necessary for her to feel secure so that whether or not she sees you, she trusts that you still exist. It is an absolutely essential psychological step for healthy development. When a child's root center is out of balance, fear that she will not survive can set in. Through your yoga sessions, you will work to release such fears. Outside the yoga sessions, you can help to develop a sense of security in your child by meeting all of her survival needs as they are expressed and reassuring your baby that you are always there for her.

The will to live is a necessity for any baby to thrive. If at any point in life the energy put out by the generator, the root center, wanes, the will to live may also wane. The exercises in this session focus on ways to stimulate the root center and fuel the will to live.

Yoga Mind

The energy of the human generator and all its natural products are the focus here. Nourishment is taken from the Earth only to be recycled to the Earth as excrement for further use. From this point of view, it is hard to imagine why some people think feces are dirty, something to be embarrassed about or laugh at, or shameful and need to be hidden. Yoga mind perceives the energy of the root center expressed as the products of the root center. As a result, yoga mind has a natural appreciation for the beauty of this process and its connection with the Earth.

Yoga Technique

To create a solid connection with the Earth and allow your baby to eventually walk naturally and without pain, it is necessary to stimulate energy flow into your baby's feet and ankles. Distributing the baby's weight evenly over the feet allows the gait to be even and balanced. Spinal alignment naturally follows from this solid foundation. The exercises in this session will prepare your baby to learn to walk with his weight evenly distributed over each foot.

The Ritual

For the root center, set up your designated yoga place with relaxing music and soft lighting. If you use incense, try tree and root scents. Put on music with a gentle beat, such as Amazonian music, or incorporate African drumbeats in the background. Colors can include any earth colors and tones.

Postures for Mom

Some pregnant women may find these movements familiar; in the West they are frequently known as Kegel exercises, but they are actually based upon yoga. In yoga they are called *mula banda,* for the movement of closing the root center.

Sit in your V or cross-legged position with your baby in any position that feels natural and try these basic movements. Both of these seated positions can be modified for stretches in one of five basic ways:

1. Seated, move forward from the waist with your hands on your knees (or supporting your baby).
2. Seated, lift your torso forward and up while taking a breath. Exhale as you roll back and down, tucking in the pelvis and keeping your hands on your knees.

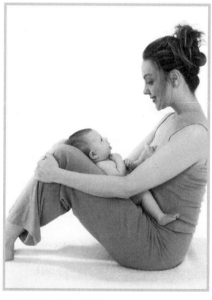

POSTURES FOR MOM

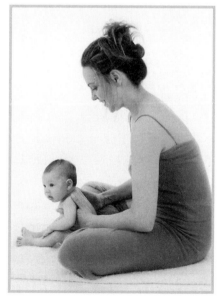

POSTURES FOR MOM

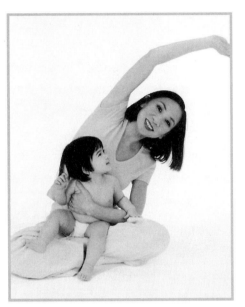

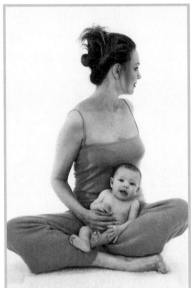

POSTURES FOR MOM   POSTURES FOR MOM

3. Seated, lean over to the side from the waist with your arm extended.
    Let your weight flow over to the right, back to the center, and over
    to your left with the buttocks planted solidly on the floor. Bring
    your nose toward your right knee, then over to your left knee.

4. Spinal twist: Sit with your legs in V formation, with the soles of
    your feet drawn in so that they're flat against each other, or cross-
    legged. Place your hands on your knees. Lengthen your back and
    twist the spine at the waist toward the right. With your left hand on
    your right knee, twist around and look over your right shoulder
    while lifting straight up from your head. Repeat the twist on the
    left side, keeping your buttocks flat on the floor. Breathe in as you
    twist, and exhale as you return to the center without letting your
    chest sink.

5. Seated, with legs bent, the soles of your feet together, and your
    hands resting on your thighs, pull up the pelvic floor by tightening

the perineal muscles, which control urine flow; practice lifting and dropping the pelvic floor by tightening and then releasing this muscle. Do this contraction, which naturally tightens the abdomen, five times, releasing your abdominal muscles after each contraction. Hold for a count of two each time.

Postures for Baby

FOOT MASSAGE

The touch used in the stimulation of the soles of the feet should be a gentle, soothing touch. Remember that a foot massage stimulates all of the baby's energy meridians and organs and is good preparation for walking. It also has been known to relieve tension in the feet and ankles. Babies' feet are warm, with elastic skin, and the toes rotate easily.

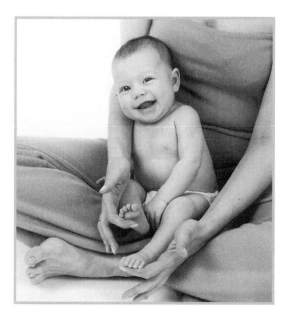

FOOT MASSAGE

1. Set the baby in any position you're comfortable working in.
2. With four fingers on top of your baby's foot and your thumb on the bottom, rub the sole of the foot with your thumb. Some babies prefer foot massage on the tops of their feet because the bottoms are too sensitive; if this is the case for your child, she may get agitated if you rub the bottoms.
3. Next, make circular movements with the cushioned part of your thumb or forefinger along the bottom of your baby's foot. Do the same for both feet.
4. Some babies like to have their feet held as well. Hold the foot at the ankle by cupping one hand underneath the ankle and the other hand over the top of the foot.
5. Take one finger of the top hand and separate each of the baby's toes one by one.
6. With your thumb, begin to massage the soles of the baby's foot in a circular movement, one foot at a time.
7. Do this for three to five minutes.

TOE SPIRAL

Moms should try this move on themselves first to get a feeling for this exercise, which nurtures the foot and allows it to develop in its most natural way.

1. With the baby on the floor between your legs, which are in a V position, lean down over her by bending from the waist and bring your head closer to her eye level. Her feet will be at your pubic bone, and her head will be away from your body.
2. With the baby centered, hold the heel of her right foot and lift it with your left hand, holding the ankle securely.
3. Take hold of all five toes in the palm of your right hand.

4. Hold the toes in a group and help her slowly rotate them clockwise. Repeat this exercise five times, resting in between repetitions.

5. Do the same move in a counterclockwise direction for five repetitions.

6. Repeat these steps using your baby's opposite foot.

ANKLE SPIRAL

Try this exercise yourself first to get a good sense of it.

1. With your baby still on her back on the floor between your V-positioned legs, or with baby in any other comfortable position, hold your baby's right calf below the knee securely but loosely in your left hand.

2. With your right hand, rotate her right foot clockwise.

3. Repeat five times, resting in between repetitions.

4. Now rotate foot counterclockwise for five repetitions.

5. Repeat on the left foot.

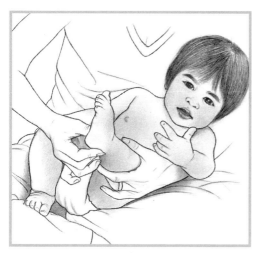

ANKLE SPIRAL

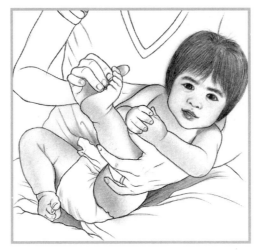

ANKLE POINT AND FLEX

ANKLE POINT AND FLEX

Try this exercise first on your own feet and feel how it brings energy to them.

1. Extend baby's right leg straight up.
2. Place the palm of your right hand flat against the sole of her flexed right foot, and tip your hand to guide her foot in toward her body (flex) and out toward you (point). This will bring energy to her feet.
3. Repeat the movement five times, resting in between repetitions.
4. Repeat on the left leg.

Postures for Babies Six to Twelve Months

Babies who are six months and older are more active and need to be positioned differently to capture their attention. Do the exercises described above, then try these additional movements while sitting cross-legged with your baby sitting in front of you. Make sure your baby is facing toward you.

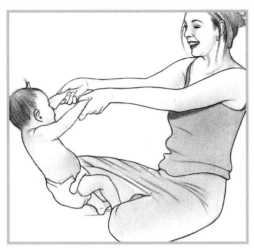

SIT AND STAND

SIT AND STAND

Grasp your baby's hands and pull her from a sitting to a standing position. She will love this.

WALKING

Now sitting V-legged, let your baby make stepping movements alongside each of your legs to stimulate walking. Use a prop (such as a chair, table, or sofa) for your baby to hold on to as she walks or let her sit and rest if that's what she prefers. Babies like to feel that they are kicking against something to feel power and express their presence.

Observations

Yoga for babies is not about exercise; it is about gentle stimulation while bonding with your baby. If your baby becomes resistant, stop and rest. You don't have any time constraints or any schedule to adhere to. Your focus should be on getting in touch with your baby's rhythms, so just relax. Place one hand on your stomach and the other hand on your baby's stomach gently. Sense her stomach gurgling and churning, as well as your own. Feel her rhythm and yours and note the similarities and differences. This is reassuring to a baby. When she has settled down, begin the exercises again. If she signals that she is tired by crying or excessive wriggling, save the rest for tomorrow.

Commonly Asked Questions

Q: My baby kicked vigorously in utero. What does this mean? Will she be hyperactive?

A: Not necessarily; she is simply expressing herself and feeling her power through resistance to another force.

Q: My baby kicks one foot and not the other. Why?

A: Perhaps your baby was positioned in utero in a way that limited his use of the other foot. Focus on evening out the energetic use of the body by stimulating the side that is not often in use through a series of lengthening and massaging movements.

Q: My baby eats a lot, and I'm afraid she'll get fat later in life. Should I limit the amount of milk in each feeding now to prevent her from becoming overweight later?

A: No need. Just feed your baby fully until she indicates that she is finished. Then gently thump the bottoms of her feet to encourage her to take the last drop needed, so that she can last longer between feedings. Discourage nibbling between meals, which confuses the schedule.

The Regenerative Center

BONDING EMOTIONALLY

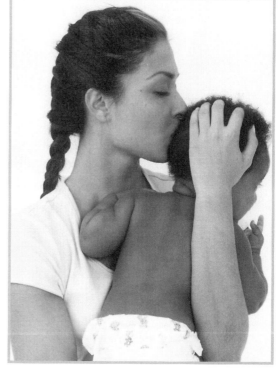

James and his mother arrived for class with his mother panting and clearly exhausted. He was a particularly large baby and from birth had been in the highest percentile for height and weight. Clearly his weight alone tired his mother out. But there was another reason for James's mom's fatigue. James wanted to be carried everywhere at all times, so that his eyes could soak up as much as possible. At three months, his curiosity outdistanced his physical ability, and he had learned how to get her to carry him everywhere so that he could see everything his body could not yet take him to. But his mother was weary and angry. James needed to work on his physical abilities to feel more able to participate in life. We were not trying to advance his development, because that comes as the brain and body mature and cannot be hurried. But we did need to find other ways to stimulate a *curious little boy. He preferred more vigorous play, even though he was only three months old. He even preferred a firmer hand during massage than did the other babies, so I gave his mother specific techniques to use with James. By having him kick his legs and bounce as strongly as he was able, he felt the power of his little legs, and even though they could not yet support his weight, he seemed less demanding of his mother. Through his Yoga Baby sessions, he got a good workout and lots of stimulation. They left him fully tired physically, and therefore less demanding. James's mother also learned to use her body more efficiently by sitting whenever she could and stimulating James in a position that suited her body.*

No matter how bitter the winter, spring still comes every year, bringing renewal to the Earth. The focus of session three is the regenerative center, which concerns bonding emotionally. The regenerative center, sometimes called the sacral center, is my personal favorite because it is the center from which most therapists like myself work. It is also the womb from which life is created. It is the symbol for mother and father. Both yin (magnetic receptive energy that draws unto itself, and is sometimes thought of as feminine) and yang (dynamic, radiating, expressive energy that flows out, and is sometimes thought of as masculine) have a home here in the sacral plexus area. While the female sex organs, the uterus and the ovaries, are considered yin, and the male sex organs, the penis and the testes, are considered yang, it is important to note that each gender has both yin and yang. Therefore I prefer not to attribute rigid feminine or masculine gender labels to these types of energies.

This center's energy brings hope, renewal, and regeneration, just as springtime brings renewed energy to the Earth. Through the sacral energy that comes with the season, the planet is transformed by green, making it alive, vibrant, and renewed. It is why we fall in love in the spring—if not with someone, then with the season itself. We are enlivened and gravitate outside, unable to contain ourselves inside because of spring fever. This is a time to expand our boundaries and to connect, and this center's focus is about connections—with food and nutrition, or with another emotionally and physically.

The regenerative center, which develops mainly between the ages of six and twenty-four months, is where we connect both with our baby and with our mate sexually. Sexual energy makes us feel young and renewed. It is the energy that allows your baby to create, continually multiplying new cells at an astounding rate so that he grows and grows unendingly into adult size. It is where your baby's assimilative organs, including the small and large intestines, are found. These organs are what make your baby able to absorb all the physical and emotional nutrients that are essential to life. With such creative forces, it's no surprise that it was the regenerative center, the center from which we create and affiliate with others, that most interested the psychoanalyst Sigmund Freud.

Because the regenerative center is the energetic center to which we turn to meet our physical and emotional needs, it also symbolizes issues with money and abundance. The color green, associated with money, also represents the sacral area. Money is sometimes described as congealed green energy—green dollar bills symbolically represent the resplendent green energy of the sacral center.

Later in life, if this energetic center is blocked, your child may have difficulty breaking these barriers and dealing with money. But when this center is balanced, your child will feel secure that all his needs will be met.

Although your baby is tiny and not able to act sexually, the regenerative center is nevertheless active. In fact, male babies may have erections and females' vaginas may lubricate shortly after birth, proving that this center is an essential tool for the growth and development of your baby even in the early years. For moms, it is the center that sends energy to heal you from the effects of the birthing process and the energy that keeps you strong for the rigors of child rearing. It is the same energy that allows you to reconnect sexually with your mate and renew your intimate connection.

Physical Purpose

The physical purpose of this center is to facilitate physical movement and exploration to connect to other things, whether objects, food, or people. The yoga movements you will practice in this session are designed to stimulate the sacral area to bring energetic strength to the assimilative organs. With this strength, your baby can move, kick, crawl, and later walk wherever he wants in order to get what he needs. Often babies who cannot yet talk express themselves emotionally through this center using robust movements. Sometimes a baby's desire to move is stronger than his physical capability to do so, and he can become frustrated. It is important to allow for the baby's physical expression of differing emotional states and for you to be attuned to these expressions so that you can be sensitive to his needs.

Psychological Purpose

It's important to help your baby learn the joys of connection so that he can experience sensate pleasures with food, parents, or caregivers. This is a highly emotional center where desire, pleasure, and need are experienced. Your baby may need milk and food to survive, but in pursuit of these needs, he may learn to enjoy your touch while nursing. He may also learn to desire greatly the smell of his mother's flesh or clothing, creating an attachment to his mother that cannot be duplicated with anyone else. Later in life, he will learn to discriminate between need and desire so that he will have some sense of proportion about his attachments. He will learn what he needs versus what he merely wants. At this young age, though, he must feel his needs being met and get pleasure from the experience.

If the permanent center is the originating spark of the work of art that is life and the root center the generator of creative energy, then the regenerative center is the artist's palette—the place where all the attachments and passions of the artist are gathered to bring pleasure. This center carries with it the possibility of feeling guilty about fulfilling one's desires for pleasure. When this center is in balance, the baby feels entitled to enjoy meeting his needs, and the child's emotional intelligence is enlivened because emotional intelligence is fostered and developed through his connection to others. Connection leads to the creation of something new or something more than what already exists.

Mothers should remember that first we nurture ourselves in order to generate enough energy to nurture another. To nurture oneself is to create a circuit of energy in which you are assured of meeting your own needs physically and emotionally. Touch is an important part of this center, because touch requires being in connection with another. We emphasize touch both for mothers who have just delivered as well as for those who are caring for their newborns. Touch is a magical treatment that stimulates the cells of the skin and even affects brain and neurological development. It is a sure way of staying connected.

Sacral energy is responsible for a mother's "falling in love" with her baby. Fathers sometimes feel left out because they sense a loss of connection to their spouse and their child as the mother's emerging link to the new baby grows more intense. If one does not understand the evolution of the process, it is easy to feel competitive and jealous. Falling in love with one's baby is a natural consequence of high energy in the sacral area. Fortunately, if the energy remains heightened, there is plenty of sacral energy for everyone, including the amount required for Mom and Dad to reconnect once the excitement of having a newborn has settled. This usually begins after the baby turns six weeks old, because the mother's body has returned to a more normal state and the baby has developed enough independence to sleep more solidly for several hours at a stretch and can tolerate being separated from Mom.

As your baby develops, he will find many physical items, such as the blanket he sleeps on or the toy he naps with, that become representative of Mom or Dad. Such objects become very meaningful and can be used to comfort your baby in your absence.

Yoga Mind

Release yourself from any preconceived notions of gender identity. Whether you have a boy or girl, use this session to indulge your baby in the joy of pleasing through touch. It is equally rewarding for both sexes. Since the regenerative center is also connected to the sexual feelings you have for your mate, you may feel anxious about allowing those feelings to emerge, but don't hold back. You can do the yoga exercises for the sacral center without worrying that they will stimulate sexual energy that you may not be ready to deal with. Sexual energy is only one band of sacral energy—others include emotional, physical, and life renewal—so performing these movements does not necessarily mean you'll feel sexual right now.

Yoga Technique

Sexual organs are located on both sides of the lower abdomen, so in performing these exercises, we try to remember to open our bodies and our babies' bodies in all directions. Move from side to side, focusing first on one side of the body, then on the other. Horizontal stretches should be executed with equal intensity in both the left and right directions. We also need to focus on the energy moving from the front to the back of the body, since sacral energy affects both areas. Lower-back pain is often the result of blocked sacral energy.

The Ritual

I like to play other cultures' fertility music during these sessions. I also love to hear birds chirping and other sounds of spring. I prefer scents that are familiar to me from growing up in Florida, such as gardenia, magnolia, azalea, and camellia. But if your background is different and different scents represent spring for you, use the ones you know. Do whatever it takes to get in touch with feeling the distinctive energy of spring. Fresh spring colors are an excellent representation of the regenerative center, and adding them—perhaps in the form of flowers, colorful pillows, or blankets—to the room where you do the following exercises will enhance your yoga atmosphere. Choose a spring-inspired CD.

Postures for Moms

PELVIC LOCK

1. Sit in a cross-legged position with your hands on your knees and the baby lying on the floor on his back in front of you.
2. Pull your stomach in, hold for four seconds, then release.
3. Repeat five times.

PELVIC LIFT

1. Reach your arms straight up overhead with your palms pressed together and your fingertips pointing up like a pencil point. This will make space for your internal organs.
2. Lift up continually, keeping your shoulders down, for five seconds at a time.
3. Release and repeat five times.

PELVIC CLOCK

1. In the same position, circle your entire upper body from pelvis to fingertips as if you were trying to draw a circle on the ceiling.
2. Do this three times clockwise, then three times counterclockwise.
3. Repeat five times.

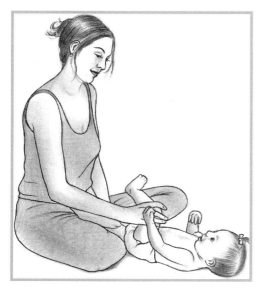

FRONTAL KNEE BENDS

Postures for Babies

FRONTAL KNEE BENDS

1. Sit cross-legged or V-legged on the floor and set your baby lying flat on her back between your legs. Gently hold her left hip flat to the floor with your right hand and use your left hand to lift the baby's right leg, bending it in at the knee toward her chest until you reach resistance. I suggest practicing this posture on the right leg first to aid the ascending colon and release gas.
2. Hold the leg there for a few seconds, then release it down to the floor by stretching it out and toward you.
3. Repeat five times, resting in between each repetition.
4. Next, stabilize the baby's right hip and raise her left leg to bend the knee into the chest, keeping the movement gentle and rhythmic.
5. Repeat five times with rests in between.

PELVIC ROLL

1. Hold both of your baby's legs in the bent-knee-to-chest position with one hand, and stabilize your baby's chest with your other hand.
2. Circle the bent legs around as if touching all the numbers on a clock.
3. Circle in one direction five times, then rest.
4. Repeat five times in the other direction, moving very slowly at all times.

SACRUM PAT

The objective is to create a circle of energy as your baby is enfolded in your hold.

1. Sit in a V-legged position and place your baby on his stomach over either knee with his arms and head extending over your knee.
2. Bend your right leg at a 45-degree angle into your chest and extend your left leg straight out. This will give you some relief from any muscle tension in the back or legs.
3. Pat the back of your baby's pelvis on the sacrum (located bewteen the waist and the buttocks) to stimulate the back of the regenerative center. Pat gently using your right hand, as you would burp your baby. He will relax and begin to enjoy the stimulation.
4. Do this for three minutes.

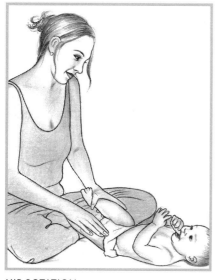

HIP ROTATION

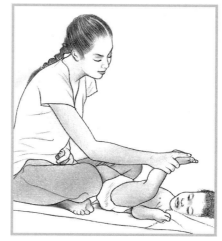

PEDAL PUSHERS

Postures for Babies Six to Twelve Months

HIP ROTATION

1. While seated with your baby lying on his back in front of you, feet toward you, gently hold her right hip flat with your left hand.
2. With your right hand, hold the baby's left thigh, keeping her knee bent.
3. Make large circles with the left thigh five times clockwise and five times counterclockwise, resting for a few seconds in between.
4. Repeat with the right leg five times in each direction.

PEDAL PUSHERS

1. Your baby should be lying on his back on the floor with his feet toward you.
2. Pedal your baby's feet, as if on a bike, for several revolutions.
3. Repeat five times, rest, and reverse direction.

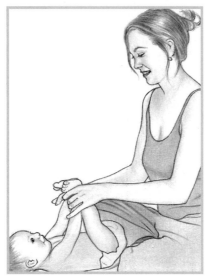

YOGIC LIFT

YOGIC LIFT

1. With your baby lying on her back and her feet closest to you, hold her feet flexed steadily in your right hand.
2. Lift her feet toward the ceiling so that her buttocks are raised off the floor.
3. Hold for a few seconds, then gently release down. Repeat five times.
4. Toe kissing is optional but highly recommended. In fact, all spontaneous shows of physical affection are to be greatly encouraged. Babies need them!

Commonly Asked Questions

Q: There is milk coming from the nipples of my newborn baby boy. Is this normal?

A: Yes, the production of a few drops of milk from the nipples of a newborn baby boy or girl is simply the result of an excess of prolactin, a pituitary hormone, that the baby received from the mother through the placenta before birth. It is perfectly normal and will abate after a few days.

Q: My baby has gas cramps. What should I do?

A: Hold the area underneath your baby's pelvis with both hands. Then remove your right hand and use it to pull his knees into his chest. Circle your baby's legs up and around, from right to left, sending an internal massage to the organs. Try this also while moving your left hand gently in a clockwise direction on your baby's tummy.

Q: My newborn has erections. Is there such a thing as too much regenerative energy?

A: No, newborn spontaneous erections are perfectly normal. This should lessen over the course of the next few days. For some babies periodic erections from tactile stimulation may occur erratically during the first year of life, but also lessen over time.

Multiple Births

Since one parent or even two parents cannot possibly provide all the physical stimulation needed by several babies, it is important to seek play equipment that allows as much leg stimulation as possible, because development of the legs and feet is needed for a child to be able to crawl, stand, and walk.

Adopted Babies

Give your baby many chances to see, hear, touch, and smell you and associate feeding and nurturing with you. If possible, feed the baby yourself, rather than delegating the job to another caregiver; also settle the baby for sleep yourself if you can. Great trust develops between baby and Mom around the transition time between wakefulness and sleep. This is prime bonding time around the regenerative center.

The Solar Plexus

BONDING EGO-TO-EGO

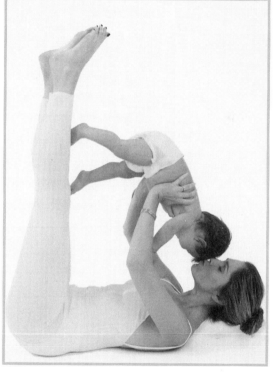

Tommy (four months old) would enter the waiting room before each class very happy and content from his walk to the center with his mother. He was at ease with his mom. However, every time he saw the other mothers and babies in the class, he would begin crying. *His solar plexus became tight and constricted, so I knew that he was afraid. I spoke with his mother about how he reacted to groups of people. It turned out that he preferred one or two people at most, but had always reacted badly to being with a larger group. She attributed this to noisiness. But our classes were very gentle, rather quiet affairs. So I suggested that she bring Tommy back on another day by himself. She did so, and Tommy was a different child. He participated in all the activities without so much as a whimper. We decided that Tommy would have Yoga Baby classes in private*

from that day forward until he adjusted to larger groups of people. Mothers sometimes laugh at me for being so sensitive to babies' reactions, but I have found that babies do try to communicate what makes them comfortable and what makes them uncomfortable, though we often don't get the communications right. There is no need to add extra stress to a baby who is in a class that is designed to increase his ability to calm himself. When Tommy is older, perhaps three or four years old, he can spend time making such adjustments. At this age, he deserves a little catering.

"Your freedom ends where my nose begins." Once your baby has developed enough energy in the permanent center to be centered spiritually, in the root center to be grounded physically, and in the regenerative center to be gratified and connected emotionally, he is ready to generate the energy of the solar plexus, which leads to a sense of himself as separate from his mother and with a will of his own. If the permanent center is the originating spark of the artwork that is life, the root center the generator that creates life energy, and the regenerative center the artist's palette, then the solar plexus is the place where the artist makes all the ego decisions about what he is creating with his paintbrush.

The solar plexus is like the brain for the body, and it is sometimes called the "second brain." It is formed before the baby's actual brain is fully developed. It is where personality development originates, and helps the baby begin to have a sense of self, feel his own power, and display his will. This is the energetic center connected with decisions about what actions the personality will take for the body. It is the place where a battle may begin between the parent's will and the baby's. In this center, the separation of self from other is inevitable.

The danger with the solar plexus center is that whenever one feels truly alone against the external world, the anxiety heightens and the solar plexus knots and closes. By acknowledging the certainty of connection to others or to something higher, one feels less alone. The solar plexus softens and begins to open, able to send and receive energy.

The first three centers develop during the first twelve to eighteen months of life. The burgeoning development of the will of the baby begins at approximately eighteen to thirty-six months of age, when the baby's individual ego is established. The solar plexus is the soft and unprotected space right below the bottom of the breastbone. It is framed on either side by the bottom of the rib cage so that it looks like a triangular soft spot, an opening to the world. The solar plexus includes the adrenal glands, the nervous system, and the organs of digestion, which are the stomach, liver, spleen, and pancreas (the last of these produces insulin and balances the body's blood sugar levels). It involves the rhythmic rise and fall of the diaphragm and the rhythm of the lungs through the breath. This forms the biorhythm of the solar plexus. This is the place where we feel "butterflies" when we're nervous.

The solar plexus is involved with digestion, what we take in and what our body uses. Initially, an infant can handle only milk, and mother's milk is usually easier than formula. Gradually the baby learns to digest more diverse foods. Eventually he learns to handle soft solid foods. The learning process for the stomach is gradual, as the energy increases to aid with digestion. The solar plexus can be a center of great empowerment when a person acts without fear, held steady by the certainty that he is not alone, but is connected to something more or something Higher. When this center is strong, it allows for freedom of action, whether to express oneself through a big belly laugh or to vocalize loudly. When we say "He dug down deep and pulled it out of himself," we are referring to the personal power drawn from his solar plexus.

On the contrary, when a person is racked with fear and unable to act, we call him "yellow-bellied." The solar plexus is blocked, making him prone to psychosomatic illness, anxiety, and phobias. The organs most identified with the solar plexus center are the adrenal glands, which are necessary because they keep one in a state of readiness to act.

This is the first center where one's will determines action, so it is related to feelings of empowerment. The products of the first chakra, feces and urine, are made without the volition of the baby, without conscious decision making. But the product of the third chakra, action, represents conscious decision making. Whatever one does or does not make with the energy of this center is an act of will.

Mothers usually become very aware of the solar plexus when a child is between two and two and a half years old, because the formerly compliant baby enters the "terrible two's," exercising his will, often arbitrarily. The child is merely trying out the power of the solar plexus center in the world. If routinely blocked in this expression, a child will develop a sense of shame about his actions and decisions. If allowed some reasonable expression of will, children may develop into empowered adults. At this stage, parents who engage in a battle of wills with their child may launch a destructive and ongoing struggle for power.

The solar plexus center, which is very responsive to the external world, is related to the baby's startle reflex. So when your baby hears a sudden, loud noise and begins to wail and tighten up, you can feel a tightening in the baby's soft solar plexus. The solar plexus is related to how the baby begins to relate to the outside world. When we feel something in our "gut," this is the center from which we are sensing.

For babies, there is such a free flow between the external world and the internal world that the separation of self from outside is not clear at the beginning. Even the mother seems an extension of the baby, as if the nipple should magically appear just because the baby feels hungry. There is a very open pathway to the stomach for baby, so that the difference between the internal and external pressure for the baby is easily adjusted through a quick spit-up or an explosive bowel discharge. From a baby's perspective, he is part of the cosmos and his spit-up and discharges are released into part of him. There is no separation. Later he will learn to control the sphincter muscle to release bowel movements at will and to close his mouth to prevent spit-up. This happens when the external and internal boundaries of himself are clear and he has enough energy to develop physical control.

The baby is learning to get energy into his body and how to live in the world. The solar plexus is a highly receptive center that provides the energy to sense what is happening externally and to take action to handle any difficulty that comes along—it is a highly yin center.

If a baby is overtired and cranky—too wired or wound up—we might check the solar plexus to calm the hyper nervous system. We use the phrase "too tightly strung" in referring to an overreactive and sensitive nervous system. Whenever a person or baby screams, it can lead to a very tight knot in the solar plexus, not just in the individual crying but also in anyone within earshot. If a mom becomes upset about a crying baby, it is best to have the mom soften and soothe her own solar plexus before attending to the baby's. Otherwise she may compound the baby's troubles. When this center opens up, one feels supported in the world, and not alone. This is a place where the certainty of connection to something or someone more is of enormous comfort both for your baby and for you.

As I mentioned earlier, you can sense the solar plexus in yourself when you let out a good old-fashioned belly laugh or a deep visceral cry. The ribs move freely, allowing these emotional expressions to come out. Another way to sense the solar plexus is to follow the old adage of alleviating your anger by holding your breath, counting to ten, and breathing out slowly. This is a simple technique to release the solar plexus and open the center to release upset feelings and receive fresh energy. It is highly effective with both children and adults.

As children take certain actions based on their will—for example, grabbing another's toy or excessively using the terms *me, my,* and *mine*—they will learn that adults think some acts are good and others are bad. But babies have a hard time understanding that one person can be capable of both good and bad. This mental task requires further mental development. To a baby, you are either all good or all bad.

I'll use my son to illustrate this concept. When he was three years old, he had a game he played with his hands as puppets. He let his right hand be a spider that did naughty, brazen acts. His left hand was a butterfly that pleased everyone and was impeccable, well-behaved, and good in all its actions. In other words, he split the two sides of his will to act into two characters. Because he had allergies, he was scheduled for one particularly intensive medical appointment at which he would receive eight injections in one sitting. The doctor suggested that five injections be given in the left arm (the left was his nonpreferred hand) and the other three be given in the right arm (his preferred hand). When my son heard this plan, he began to wail, "Not the butterfly." I knew instinctively the butterfly could not handle the terror of the injections. He needed the tough spider in order not to be overwhelmed by fear. So I told the doctor that my son would take all eight injections in the right arm. He objected, but my son did not. Finally the doctor, mystified, acquiesced to our request. The spider sat calmly for all eight injections and the butterfly danced about excitedly watching the whole experience. My son never cried and never complained later. I had managed to do what I recommend to all parents: I had gotten synchronized with my son's solar plexus, and I had intuited what was needed for him to release his fear and face a frightening situation bravely.

Physical Purpose

Because the adrenal glands are on both sides of the body, it is necessary to create greater flexibility in the spine through a twisting motion to each side with equal power. This opens up the solar plexus, allowing more freedom of movement.

The solar plexus often gets involved with all sorts of psychosomatic disorders that affect the breath, such as anxieties and phobias. A prime example is asthmatic reactions. When a child has allergies, she is often susceptible to asthma, which can be a frightening experience for both parent and child. My experience with this condition is with children in the Center. First you must clear your own solar plexus of the fear that your child cannot breathe and may die; you can do this by first slowing your own breath and breathing as deeply as you can into the belly. This not only calms you, but also serves as a model to help slow and deepen your child's breath. Once you have calmed yourself, turn your attention to your child. I have found that children respond best to lying flat on the floor with your right hand over the knotted area at the solar plexus and your left hand underneath your child at the same level. Use your mind to create heat in your hands, and imagine sending heat from one hand to the other, penetrating your child's body. In this way, you can release a cramped spot (a heating pad is not nearly as effective). Gradually the diaphragm will start to lower, thereby creating a greater space for the lungs to expand into. Keep your breath even, deep, and slow to be effective. This should work until you can get the child to take the necessary medication or, if need be, get to the hospital. This same technique of releasing the solar plexus will work for your child if she becomes panicked.

Psychological Purpose

It is important to reduce fear and anxiety in order to help a baby develop a strong and solid sense of his own will. It is also important for your will to be aligned with that of your baby to ensure greater harmony; this means less stress and fewer battles of the will between you. At numerous times in your child's life, you will need to know the status of the solar plexus so that you can determine how best to soothe, protect, and empower her.

Yoga Mind

Babies do not make bad decisions; they act neither good nor bad. They are only learning to act, and need not be ashamed of either action or inaction. They make no wrong decisions, since they are simply testing out their own will and expressing the solar plexus at the same time. We adults need to guide children into what we consider appropriate behavior as they mature, but without shaming. To shame a child is to inhibit his behavior by mocking, making fun of, ridiculing, humiliating, or punishing him for behavior that you do not like. This may inhibit the unwanted behavior, but the child will carry the emotional baggage for a long time, and it will block the energy of the solar plexus center. When we guide a child's behavior with love and understanding, we can achieve the desired goal without being destructive to his development and expression of will.

Yoga Technique

Since the adrenal glands sit on both sides of the body, as mentioned earlier, focus on moving the baby's body in two opposite sideways directions with equal force and intensity so that the adrenal glands are given more room to open the solar plexus area. For example, as the baby's lower body is turned sideways in one direction, hold the upper portion with equal intensity in the opposite direction, creating a swivel action around the vertical axis of the spine. This results in the flexibility so necessary for an open solar plexus and your baby's healthy personality.

The Ritual

The wind instruments seem most related to the solar plexus. Opt for action music, even military marches, played by wind instruments. One example is Scottish bagpipes, played as soldiers were being encouraged to exhibit valor in battle. In order to play the bagpipes, one would have to have an open solar plexus, and also the sound of the bagpipes encourages others to have an open solar plexus—in other words, to exercise their strong will to fight and be victorious.

Postures for Moms

As you perform these exercises, try to feel how your solar plexus is tied to the rhythm of your breath. Feel your baby's rhythm, then match it with your own. You can feel the rise and fall of your own diaphragm as your lungs contract and then expand. Your baby's diaphragm, too, lowers, and then the lungs expand to fill the space.

THE SEATED SPIRAL TWIST

The seated spiral twist helps keep the spine flexible and opens the solar plexus. Place the baby comfortably nearby.

1. Keeping your spine straight, sit with your weight distributed evenly over both sit bones (ischial tuberosities).
2. Fold your left leg into your buttocks with your left heel pressed up against your right buttock.
3. Bring the right leg over the left leg and place the right foot close to the left knee on the floor.
4. Place your right hand behind you with your fingertips touching the floor and turn your body and head to the right.

5. Cradle your left arm around your right leg so your left elbow is touching your right knee and the fingertips of your left hand are on the floor.

6. Hold the posture for a few breaths, lifting your spine to the ceiling with each inhalation and extending the stretch farther with each breath.

7. Reverse the entire position to the other side, with the right leg folded in and the left leg folded over the right leg, spiraling to the left side.

8. Repeat five times on each side.

SEATED BACKWARD ARM LIFT

1. With your baby lying on her back in front of you, sit with your legs crossed in front at the pubic bone, straight arms placed behind you with palms on the floor, and your chest open so that your shoulder blades practically touch. This forces an opening in the front of the body to give more room to the internal organs and to open the solar plexus.

2. Inhale and exhale deeply in this position while lifting your arms, but not the shoulders, higher. Make sure you are sitting squarely over the sit bones.

CAT STRETCH

This move will help you gain flexibility in your spine and release your lower tailbone area.

1. Place your baby on a mat on her back with her toes pointing toward you.

2. Place your right hand to the right of the baby's head and your left hand to the left of the baby's head. Be sure your hands are shoulder width apart.

3. Place your right knee to the right of the baby's foot and the left knee

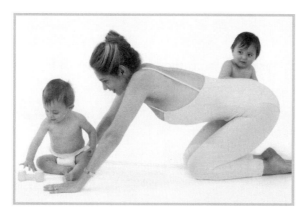

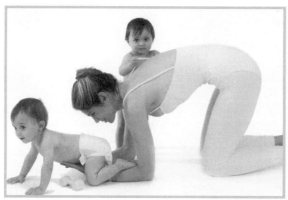

CAT STRETCH

to the left of the baby's foot so that your baby is directly under you, as if protected by a four-cornered structure.

4. Then make a flat table of your back so that someone could place a cup on it.

5. On an inhale, simulate the form of a cat by first arching your back so that the buttocks are pushed up.

6. After a count of five inhales and five exhales, return to table position. Repeat this movement five times.

7. On an exhale, create a round back so that the buttocks move toward the floor. Your pelvis is thrust forward.

8. Hold for five breaths, then return to the neutral or table position. Repeat five times.

9. Look back to your left for one breath, then look back to your right for one breath, and finally return to neutral position.

If your babies are mobile, let them move about the space observing and exploring as you move. Stay energetically connected and they will not venture very far from mom.

REST TIME

Once you have completed these exercises, move away from your baby into Child's Pose. This is a time to rest.

1. To form Child's Pose, first kneel on your mat, then sit back on your heels.

2. Next, fold your upper body over your knees and drop your forehead to the floor.

3. Place your arms next to your legs on the floor, with hands facing up and fingers pointing toward your toes.

4. Hold the position as you breathe deeply for several minutes to completely relax yourself.

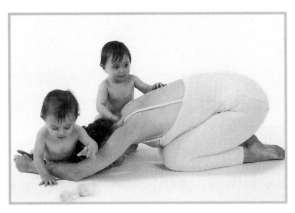

REST TIME

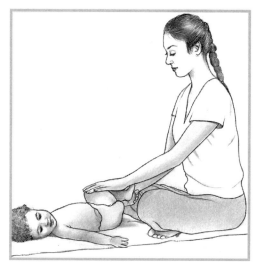

SPINAL TWIST

Postures for Baby

SPINAL TWIST

1. Place your baby on the mat so that her feet are near your pubic bone.
2. With your left hand, raise both her legs together, bend the knees, and bring the legs up in a bent position toward the chest.
3. Place your right hand flat on the floor next to your baby's cheek.
4. Without letting go of her legs, use your right hand and slowly move her head to the left while simultaneously using your left hand to gently press her legs to the right side so that they are touching the floor.
5. Get her attention by dropping your head to the floor to face her turned cheek so she can see you.
6. Hold this position for several seconds, then return to the starting position.
7. Alternate sides by changing hands and twisting the baby to the opposite side.

8. Repeat five times on each side.

9. Return the baby's legs to the down position. If your child is unable to twist in both directions, then do a variation by moving her legs to one side while holding the opposite shoulder down.

PRONE LEG LIFTS LYING ON STOMACH

This exercise can be done with both legs or with one leg at a time.

1. Your baby should be lying on her stomach on the floor in front of you while you are seated in a half-lotus position (cross-legged with each heel sitting on top of the opposite knee).

2. Put your left hand on your baby's back and slip your right hand under the baby's right thigh and knee.

3. Slide your right hand forward to the foot, lengthening the leg and lifting it up an inch (not more), then bringing the leg back down to the floor in one smooth motion.

4. Repeat five times.

5. Now repeat the entire exercise on the other leg. Do five repetitions.

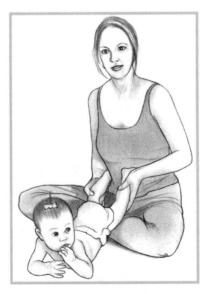

PRONE LEG LIFTS LYING ON STOMACH

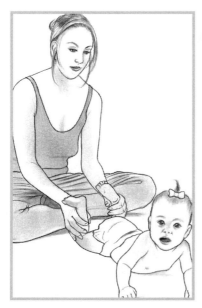

KNEE BENDS LYING ON STOMACH

KNEE BENDS LYING ON STOMACH

This exercise can be done with both legs or one at a time.

1. Keep the baby in the same position as she was in for the last exercise.
2. Put your left hand on your baby's back and slip your right hand under the baby's right thigh and knee.
3. Slide your right hand forward to the foot and lift the leg up an inch, keeping the knee bent. Then bring the leg back down to the floor.
4. Repeat five times.
5. Now repeat the entire exercise on the other leg. Do five repetitions.

Postures for Babies Six to Twelve Months

The point of the following movements is to do a slight back bend so that the spine is stimulated in the direction opposite from its normal bends.

THE LOCUST

The locust and half bow positions are both powerful convex positions that bend the spine inward. This affects the lumbar portion of the spine and provides increased flexibility. Psychologically, these positions are beneficial for opening up the energetic channels for the free expression of the will or the individualized ego, which becomes predominant from eighteen months to three years of age.

1. Lay the baby on his stomach in front of you with his hands wherever they are comfortable and his head turned to one side.
2. You should be seated in a half-lotus position (see Prone Leg Lifts exercise, page 88, for an explanation).
3. Move your hands under the baby's ankles to hold them.

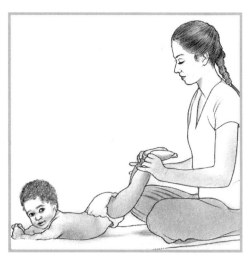

THE LOCUST

4. Gently lift his ankles, legs, and hips off the ground. Hold for as long as your baby allows this, then gently release and lower the hips, legs, and ankles to the floor.

5. Repeat five times.

HALF BOW

1. Your baby should be lying on her stomach in front of you with her hands over her head. Sit in a half-lotus position with the baby's feet closest to you.

2. Pull her arms together behind her with your right hand.

3. Take hold of both of the baby's hands with your right hand to lift the baby slightly up and back.

4. With your left hand holding the baby's feet, bring them closer to the hands so that feet and hands are as close as possible behind the baby's back.

5. Hold for five seconds, then release.

6. Repeat five times; make sure to make a game of this by talking to your baby to encourage cooperation.

Commonly Asked Questions

Q: How do I get my baby to twist in the spiral twist exercise?

A: It is not difficult to get the lower portion of the body to twist, because you will have the knees held in your hand to move to one side or the other. However, your baby may resist your turning her head in the opposite direction. I find it is helpful to use a toy to encourage the baby to look in the given direction as you shift the hips in the opposite direction. If the baby is just too stiff to turn, do not fight the resistance; simply revert to the variation of the exercise in which you hold the shoulders flat on the floor as the lower body is twisted.

Q: When my baby is on her stomach, can she breathe?

A: Yes, but be sure to allow her head the freedom to turn to either side. If she is very young, she may not have the strength to lift her head from the mat, interfering with easy breathing.

Q: If I do knee bends with my baby on her back, why should I do knee bends with my baby on her stomach, too? Aren't these the same exercises?

A: Both versions are necessary because you are stimulating a different energetic center with each. Knee bends on the back (see Frontal Knee Bends exercise, page 69) affect the regenerative center primarily, while knee bends on the stomach (see Knee Bends Lying on Stomach exercise, page 89) have more of an effect on the solar plexus. Most yogic positions work the vertebrae in one direction and then reverse the bend to work the vertebrae in the opposite direction to maintain flexibility. These two positions are an example of working the spine in two different directions, forward and backward, so that the body's energy use is balanced.

Q: Can the twist harm my baby?

A: Only if you force it when you reach resistance. A baby may initially not prefer this movement because it is new and unusual. Psychological resistance can be worked around through encouragement and distraction, but physical resistance is not to be pushed. Stop when you feel your baby's physical resistance.

Q: If the spine is rigid and refuses to be turned, does this signify a powerful solar plexus?

A: No, an open, powerful solar plexus suggests great spinal flexibility, not rigidity.

Fathers

Sometimes I have had a father or a mother, but more frequently a father, be concerned that a male child not be coddled too much. The concern seems to be that life is difficult and male children especially need to be ready to meet the demands they will encounter. In one particular class, a father tended to give little attention to his son when he cried, although the father was in every other way extraordinarily attentive and loving with his son. When I asked the father about why this might be so, he indicated that he wanted his son to be tough and not a "candy ass"; he felt that paying less attention to his son's crying would achieve this goal. I tried to explain that what he was doing would not create a tough, strong child, but instead a child who, when afraid, knew the world would be of no help and that he was truly alone. If the child held his position, it would be out of fear, not strength. I told the father that an obstinate will is one factor in some back injuries; what happens is that such people maintain a rigid posture and will not back down. I also explained that to allow a child to feel unsupported emotionally and then to judge him harshly for emotional outbursts shamed the child and thereby inhibited the child's empowerment. My motto is "Never shame a child for action or inaction."

Caregivers

Although the task of caring for a child is easier with one who is very agreeable and cooperative, please remember that all children who are growing into healthy adults should at some time exercise their will. This is how they learn to be in the world. It does not mean that you are not a completely good caregiver if the child does so. A totally compliant child is not the ideal.

Multiple Births

Fear is contagious. When one baby is startled, chances are that others will begin to cry also. To get a handle on a problem that seems in danger of getting completely out of control, try comforting them one at a time by separating them from the group, even removing them to another room if possible. Begin by comforting the initially startled baby, because he will be the most difficult to settle, then take the second, third, and so on, until they are all gradually settled. Otherwise you may be in for a long crying spell.

Adopted Babies

In the womb, babies become accustomed to the sounds and vibrations of their mother. When they are taken at whatever age after birth to a whole new set of people with different sounds, smells, touches, and vibrations, they often display very obvious reactions to these unfamiliar stimuli. This can lead the adopted baby to be initially wary, hesitant, and sometimes afraid. All this is seen in both the child's behavior and the status of the solar plexus. It is extremely important to allow a newly adopted baby much time to adjust, without any expectations from the adoptive parents. Some babies adjust quickly and some slowly. But an adoptive parent's patience is the best predictor of a successful transition for the adopted baby to its new home and new parents. It is here that generous doses of love and patience are essential.

The Heart Center

BONDING EMPATHETICALLY

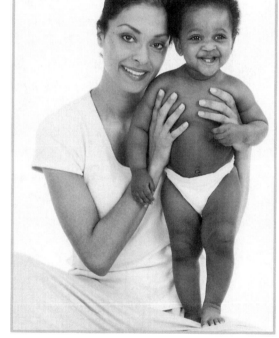

Eric was brought to class by a mother suffering from fibromyalgia, which she said prevented her from being able to pick up her two-month-old baby. In fact, since his birth, she had rarely picked him up or touched him. His basic needs were provided for by a nanny. In class, either I or one of the other mothers picked Eric up and walked him through all the steps of the exercises for his mom. She enjoyed the yoga parts for herself but was far less interested in the yoga portions for Eric. She stayed for the first four sessions, dealing with the first four energetic centers. But when we got to the fifth energetic center, the heart, she was clearly dismayed. It became painfully obvious to the other mothers that not only was she unable to participate with her baby physically, she actually did not wish to participate with him. In fact, it was hard to see that she liked him at all. Eric had *learned to manage on his own rather well. He did not look to his mother for much of anything. She even had him drink his bottle propped by pillows completely independently, despite the fact that he could not yet hold a bottle. Somehow little Eric managed with all this. The other mothers were quick to offer to do more for Eric. After the fifth session, on the heart chakra, his mother announced that she had decided not to attend any additional Yoga Baby classes and would instead focus on her own yoga separately. I accepted her decision, but I was very sad for Eric. I made sure to send him as much of my own heart energy as I could muster before they departed. I do not know what happened to Eric, but I always wonder about him, and hope someone is providing love for him. Some mothers warm up slowly to their babies, and it is possible that Eric's mom will warm up to him in time.*

The heart, like the sun, radiates the invisible substance that sustains and vitalizes a life. The focus of this session is the heart energetic center. An open heart center, like the sun, is always shining no matter what you do, whether you request it or not, and whether you appreciate it or not. It requires nothing of you. As the sun sustains the life of everything within the galaxy, a radiating heart sustains the life within its energetic boundaries. Unconditional love, the most remarkable of human potentials, was exemplified in the lives of some notable figures, including Mother Teresa, Mahatma Gandhi, Jesus Christ, and Princess Diana, who wished to be known as the "queen of hearts." The heart energy connected you to your baby before his birth and nourished him in utero. It is that same heart energy that will care for him throughout his life, vitalizing and sustaining him through all the emotional upheavals and vicissitudes he will inevitably encounter.

If the permanent center is the originating spark of the artist's life, the root center the generator of artistic energy, the regenerative center the artist's palette, and the solar plexus the decision-making center, then the heart center is the place where all the artist's connections of relationships, colors, shapes, and themes are gathered for potential expression. It is the empty canvas of life with endless possibilities.

Your baby arrives ready to radiate. You may send heart energy directly to your baby immediately, but at the outset your baby sends heart energy less discriminately and less personally. At first, your baby's heart energy is there for anyone and everyone with whom he comes in contact. It is extraordinary to watch how a baby can melt the hardest of hearts. A baby's heart energy changes those around him. People become happier, kinder, more loving. If a baby is present, most everyone will make some effort to communicate with him, whether by making eye contact, making faces, saying "coochy-coo," or picking him up. Who can resist a baby's charms? Perhaps this is why advertisements featuring babies are so successful.

Your baby will connect to you initially using his lower three chakras. But as he grows older, your ability to radiate love to him will determine a great deal about how he will radiate love to you and others. He must first be loved and accepted unconditionally in order to get the heart center activated; only then can he show love to you specifically. Self-acceptance is the prerequisite for acceptance of others. For a child, this becomes possible usually in the preschool years at between approximately three and seven years of age. Your baby will learn that he has a right to be loved and therefore a right to love. Thus, the heart center is where deeper, more intimate relationships—like family and peer relationships—are formed. This center is about relating for reasons beyond personal gratification; it is also about establishing your baby's social identity and self-esteem.

The heart energetic center is at the center of the chest and stands squarely in the middle, between the three lower energetic centers (primarily related to earthly matters) and the three higher energetic centers (more focused on spiritual concerns). Some call the heart chakra the great divider, but I call it the great unifier because it draws everything together in one central spot where love is the glue that holds all together.

The season most clearly related to the heart is the Christmas/Hanukkah season. It makes perfect sense that the colors of green and red would mark the occasion. Red symbolizes the heart, just like at Valentine's Day, because the actual heart is filled and replenished with rich, nourishing, red blood that feeds every cell of the body and takes vital breath filled with oxygen to every cell. The color green is symbolic of regeneration. So the spiritual significance of the season is the renewal of oneself into one's spiritual self. It is like a rebirth. In fact, during this time we make a point of showing love to all those whom we owe some expression of appreciation, whether they be family, friend, or acquaintance. It is a beautiful time of union.

The key word for the heart center is *expansion.* The lower three centers keep your baby tied to his individual self. The heart center is the first center that allows the individual ego to be expanded beyond oneself. Just as the first three centers establish boundaries, this chakra expands those boundaries. The heart is the hearth that draws everyone into the home and into the kitchen to see what is cooking on the stove. It is the force that guides us out of self-centered interests, opening up the possibility for real love; it encourages us to consider how others feel and what is good for them. Your baby will not be able to do that right away. You will have to be the radiating sun for your baby, and he will have to soak up all that radiating love. Love is a way to grow beyond yourself and expand your own boundaries; one day your child will be able to return love and express it to you.

The first time your child says "I love you" is sheer ecstasy for most parents. But the child must have an "I" before he can say, "I love you." He must have activated the four lower energy centers, developed a sense of ego, and then activated the fifth center to feel "I love you" and express it. At first, before your baby has words, this love may come as a kiss from the heart. Some call this a "soul kiss." I'll never forget my son's first heartfelt kiss. We were at church and he was sitting on my lap facing me. In the midst of the music, he felt moved to give me a mouth-to-mouth kiss with his little arms locked around my neck in a death grip. He was unwilling to let go for what seemed to be several minutes. I was literally trapped against the pew by a heartfelt kiss. I could not release myself from his embrace, and I felt slightly silly with the other parishioners watching the unending kiss. He could not yet talk, but for the first time, he was showing the concept of "I love you." It was quite a surprise and a magical moment.

At a higher level of development, as a person matures emotionally, the heart center is related to empathy and compassion. With babies we begin to build the way for bonding empathetically by being empathetic with them. We call this mirroring their emotions. Before language develops, we can share their mood. To empathize with a baby is to feel as the baby feels. As they cry, we sometimes mirror their upset to show we understand, not to mock them but to connect with them. When language develops, we put words to the mirroring to show we understand: "You are feeling sad today." "What a happy boy you are!" "Could anyone smile a bigger smile than you?" Empathetic bonding is the hallmark of a good psychotherapist and of a doctor with a good bedside manner. Bonding empathetically ensures that others won't feel alone. When we provide it for a baby, he grows calm and feels assured.

Love is an invisible link that exerts incredible influence and power. A baby can certainly fall in love with his mother, and actually a baby even falls in love with Mother Earth. This connection to the planet leads to a will to be here and a desire to enjoy the fruits of the planet, whether food, surroundings, or weather. Heart energy is not about self; it is about the loved one.

In the Yoga Baby program, we deal with bonding, connecting you in love to your baby. Sometimes the heart energy bond is so strong between you and your baby that it leads to jealousy from your mate or the baby's siblings. The father can help at this time by giving more than he will be receiving from his mate. The father is a natural source of heart energy and can replenish the energy that Mom gives to her child. Moms who breast-feed deliver milk along with heart energy. This milk is filled with thymus gland immunities to protect their babies and help build the strength of their own thymus gland. Moms can be so busy giving from this center that their shoulders can slope over and their chests may become caved in. An exhausted heart chakra needs replenishment of energy from loving family and friends. Moms need to make that connection and open up their hearts to receive their love.

Physical Purpose

Once it has developed, your baby's heart must pump the life force until he returns his borrowed cells to the planet. The heart and the lungs are allied and related to the heart chakra. The heart center includes the thymus gland, which develops in the first few years of a baby's life to help him learn how to live in the world and develop immunity to diseases.

Because the heart and lungs are associated with the heart center, we use movements that help baby and mom open the chest cavity, both front and back, to allow more space for the internal organs, which in turn permits easy breathing. When the physical chest cavity is less constricted, it opens the pathway for clear energetic connections.

Psychological Purpose

The beautiful, unifying heart energy is there for you to help your baby feel loved unconditionally, to connect heart to heart, and to bond empathetically. This means that you will be able to intuit what your baby is feeling, whether spoken or not. This is essential for being able to meet the emotional needs of your baby. It is a parental skill essential for the lifetime of a child. To be loved unconditionally means that your baby is valued just by virtue of his existence, no matter what he does with his life. It is not necessary for your baby to achieve or attain anything for you to feel love for him. This is the purest form of love from parent to child and it is the source from which your child feels self-acceptance and later can provide love to another. It is the essence of what glues people together and allows them to weather many storms. It is what held my family together through our trials and tribulations. In my opinion, it is pure magic.

Yoga Mind

Love is selfless. Try to remove all your expectations of what your baby is supposed to be now or in the future. You have only one day—this day— to make this moment just about the two of you. You should have no expectations, except to connect heart to heart in a bond of unconditional love.

Yoga Technique

To be able to work in the heart center requires recognizing all the self-protective ways we avoid emotional or physical vulnerability. Here's a physical example of protection of the heart we use every day: The armpit is a protected and guarded area and a direct route to the heart. If you raise your arms up overhead with the armpits exposed, see how much more vulnerable you feel than if you fold your arms across your chest to close the armpits.

The Ritual

You might try the scent of cypress for comfort. I particularly like the scent of winter evergreen trees. The flowers of love, such as iris, rose, and magnolia, are all appropriate. The colors I always think of in connection with the heart center are red and green. For background music, try a soft drumbeat to match the beat of the heart, or the sounds of a blazing fire, evoking images of the hearth warming the home. Any other music used should be flowing and romantic—violins are a favorite.

Postures for Moms

CHEST EXPANSION

With baby nearby in a comfortable position, begin this movement.

1. In a seated half-lotus position, lace your fingers behind your back, straighten your arms, lift your chest up at the same time you lift your hands up behind your back and breathe five times. Be sure not to arch your back and try to keep your spine aligned during this exercise.
2. Extend and stretch, then release. Do five repetitions.

CAT STRETCH

1. With your baby lying on the floor in front of you, feet close to you, position yourself on your hands and knees with your hands on the floor, one on each side of your baby's body, under the arms.
2. Sit back on your heels and stretch your back, leaving your arms where they are and dropping your head to your chest.
3. Extend back up until you're on your knees and stretch your back up to the ceiling like a cat, then flatten it straight.
4. Repeat five times.

HEART TO HEART

1. With the baby still vertically in front of you, sit back on your heels with your arms stretched out in front of you. Lean forward, supporting your weight on your elbows.
2. Shift your weight forward onto your knees and place your hands under your baby's back and neck.
3. Turn your head sideways and press your ear to your baby's heart. Hold for thirty seconds.
4. Repeat five times, turning your head to the other side each time.
5. Next, with your hands still supporting your baby's neck and back, shift your weight forward on your elbows so that you're leaning over the baby and lower your heart to your baby's heart. Hold for thirty seconds and release.
6. Repeat five times.

Postures for Baby

THE HOME STRETCH

Because a baby's hands are often in a clenched position, it is important to open them up and stretch them with a gentle massage of the palms. Babies must be able to open their hands in order to crawl.

1. Grasp one of your baby's hands between your thumb and fingers and gently massage the center of the palm with your thumb while your other hand is uncurling and stretching out the fingers of the same hand.
2. Slide your hand over the baby's hand as you stretch the fingers so that they are slightly bent back. Do this for thirty seconds.
3. Holding the baby's hand between your thumb and fingers again, use your other hand to stretch each finger individually, massaging each finger from bottom to top one at a time.

4. Take one finger of your hand that is doing the stretching and trace the perimeter of the baby's hand and each finger so that all fingers are gently separated.

5. With your massaging hand, hold the baby's wrist between your thumb and finger and rotate it gently from side to side.

6. Repeat on the opposite hand and wrist.

ARM LENGTHENING

1. With the baby on his back on the floor in front of you, allow him to grasp your hands.

2. See if you can move the baby's arms straight up to his head, one at a time, stretched in a lengthening movement, then down to his sides again.

3. Repeat five times.

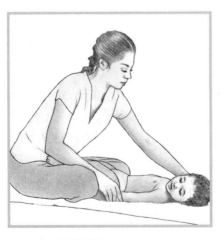

ARM LENGTHENING

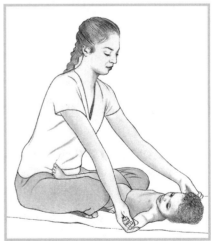

CHEST EXPANSION

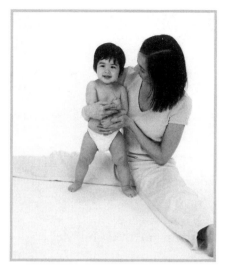

CHEST EXPANSION

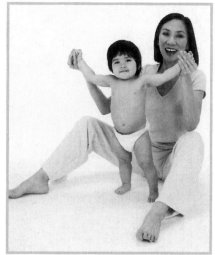

CHEST EXPANSION

CHEST EXPANSION

1. With your baby on his back on the floor, let him grasp the forefinger or thumb of each hand with each of his hands and close your hands over his.
2. Then, as he inhales, stretch his arms out to the side, opening the rib cage.
3. As he exhales, cross his arms snugly over his chest to close the rib cage.
4. Repeat five times.

Note: This exercise can also be done with your baby standing up.

A PAT ON THE BACK

1. Pick up your baby and hold him over your left shoulder as if you're burping him. Feel the baby heart to heart and feel the rhythm of his breath.
2. Gently pat the back of the baby, which is the back of the baby's heart center.
3. Do this five times.

SOCIAL RESPONSE TO MOTHER'S IMAGE

1. Hold your baby up facing you so that you are in his full view.
2. Begin to stimulate a social response by cooing to your baby or smiling. Encourage social interaction.

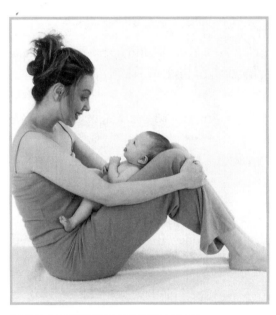

SOCIAL RESPONSE TO MOTHER'S IMAGE

Postures for Babies Six to Twelve Months

TWISTING RIGHT AND LEFT

1. Seated in a V position with your legs bent slightly, hold your baby up heart to heart.
2. Extend your arms to move the baby away from you and return him to your heart-to-heart position.
3. Rock your body from left to right five times.

BABY SIT-UPS

1. Sit in the lotus position on the floor with your baby sitting on the floor in front of you and facing you.
2. Hold his fingers and help him pull himself up to a standing position.
3. Then let him lower himself back down on his buttocks.
4. Continue as long as your baby is interested.

Commonly Asked Questions

Q: This is my second baby and I don't feel the same way I did about my first. How can I connect heart to heart when I feel this way?

A: Connecting heart to heart is not about comparing love. First you must remove all expectations of how it is supposed to be or how you are supposed to feel. Just allow your own heart energy to radiate freely, and then allow yourself to sense the baby's heart rhythms. Give yourself plenty of time to let your natural feelings develop. Don't set any expectations or create any timetables.

Q: My baby does not like when I open her arms to the sides. What should I do?

A: Start with extra time on the hand massage. Do not force her to move her arm out if she resists. Just massage the length of the side of the body from armpit to hip and the length of the arm next to the body. Gently open the hand, then let it close. Repeat several times before proceeding with the exercise.

Q: I love my baby so much; I would prefer to be dead if I were to lose my baby. Is this a normal way to feel?

A: That is a view held by many new parents, an expression of the intensity of their feeling for their babies. All relationships change, however. A baby continues to grow and go through many stages of development, and ultimately must leave your home and live on his own. You are preparing your baby to leave you, just as you did when you held him in utero. You fed him until he was ready to be delivered to this world and to live apart from you. Enjoy your intense closeness now, but remember that everything changes.

Fathers

Many men complain of having sired a baby out of love only to be displaced in their wife's eyes by the baby. They are sometimes extremely resentful. It is true that babies are easy to fall in love with, but it is also true that the connection between the mother and father is the foundation for the entire family. If the union of the mother and father is not nurtured, even with all the excitement of a new baby, then the family will have emotional difficulty. So I suggest to fathers that they try to be patient for the first three months of a new baby's life and to find their own ways of bonding with the baby. However, I also suggest that mothers try to find ways to reconnect to their husbands, to include them, and to find special time for them. Even if a couple can find time together only after the baby goes to sleep, it is important to mark that time as a time reserved just for the two of them. Many mothers have to be reminded to do this. After the first few months, it gets easier to plan a day that includes time for Mom and Dad together.

Caregivers

The pain of any loving caregiver is the worry about having to give up the baby when the family's child-care needs change. All relationships, even that of a mom and her baby, come to an end. Feel free to love as freely as you wish each day, because you have only today to connect with a baby. If you love a baby less today, it does not lessen the sense of loss when you are no longer caring for the baby. You cannot love a baby too much; there is no such thing.

Multiple Births

How does a parent have enough love for so many babies? I always say that love is like popcorn: You pop a few kernels and they just seem to create more and more, continually expanding. The more seeds you have, the more corn you have to pop. Just open your heart and let it radiate for all the little ones with whom you have been blessed. In the process, accept all the help that is offered—you'll need it.

Adopted Babies

If you adopted your baby through some channel that delayed your baby's arrival for several weeks, months, or even longer after her birth, please be patient. You do not necessarily know what the baby experienced in those early days, even if someone endeavors to tell you. Only the baby knows what she experienced and how it impacted her. Keep your patience and let her heal from the experience and the loss of it before you expect her to be happy to be with you. Thanks to all your patience and open heart energy, in time she will return the love.

The Throat Center

BONDING EXPRESSIVELY

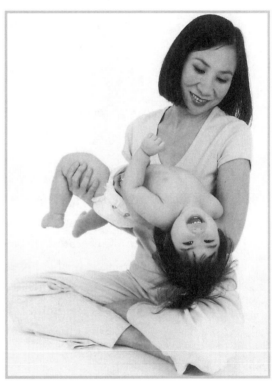

Dressed like a little angel in pink and white, Jenny, at six months, was a meticulously cared-for child. Her mother was obviously delighted in her, but her father felt that because Jenny could not yet talk, he could not understand what she wanted and did not know how to deal with her. This is a common problem for both mothers and fathers. When Jenny and her father arrived I decided to spend the entire session in silence to help him see that he understood more from nonverbal communication than he thought he did. Instead of giving verbal directives, I took his hands and put them on his baby, letting him feel her heart, her lungs, and her other organs. As we quieted, she seemed to become more vocal. Perhaps she had always been this vocal, but maybe everyone had been so busy talking that her vocalizations were not fully heard. We just listened and did yoga*

softly and quietly together. Her dad spent nearly a full hour with me until Jenny fell asleep, exhausted. She had made a variety of sounds and expressed a variety of feelings. As she slept, I began to talk to her dad, discussing his observations and his reactions to her vocalizations. He had many ideas about what Jenny was communicating, and all were very similar to what I thought Jenny was saying. We discussed bonding before a baby is fully verbal and how important it is for both the mom and the dad to find a way to do so. He left a more confident man, and he has kept up with his own yoga as well.

The focus of the sixth session is the throat energetic center, a highly creative center where communication takes place. Just as no two snowflakes are the same, no two babies are the same. The puzzle of your baby's particular uniqueness will be discovered through the baby's throat center, her expression of self. The throat emanates vibrations, which become sounds or words; these, along with gestures, are what we use to communicate with one another. The throat center includes the narrow passageway of the neck and larynx, the voice box, from which one communicates the ideas from one's head and the sensations from one's body—sometimes called the mind/body connection because it is the only way for one to express what one thinks, feels, and senses. It is the connection between the inside world and the outside world, the physical connection of your baby's head or mind to her body. It is the key center from which you learn about your baby's experiences in life and through which her creativity is expressed.

The throat center, which undergoes its greatest development between the ages of six and twelve years, includes self-expressions ranging from the mundane, such as daily conversation, to the refined, such as performance in the arts. It allows us to create a balance between integrating ideas from the head with the impulses of the body. This narrow gateway, located at the top of the spinal column where it fits into the head, has little flesh and no protective bone surrounding it. In a sense it is like the eye of a needle—so small, yet so necessary for creating a stitch.

The throat center includes the lower part of your baby's face, encompassing the nose, ears, sinuses, jaws, teeth, mouth, tonsils, tongue, and neck. It includes the thyroid and parathyroid glands, which are responsible for hormones that affect body growth and mental development. The neck muscles that will allow your baby to hold up her head do not develop sufficient strength until about one to two months of age.

If the permanent center is the originating spark of the work of art that is life, the root center the generator of creative energy, the regenerative center the artist's palette, the solar plexus the decision-making center, the heart center the canvas, then the throat center is the creative act—the artist's particular brush strokes, patterns, and themes that make up a life. It is that moment of truth when the artist takes a brush to an empty canvas.

From the first breath she took, your baby made a choice to live, because to breathe is to live and to live is to breathe. From the first to the last breath, we are given this choice. Every exhalation, even that of a baby who is not yet able to talk, is an expression of self. A baby takes her initial breath of vital air and expresses herself with a cry as soon as she is born, activating the throat center and clearing the airway of mucus. Healthy babies cry out to expand the lungs. Babies that do not are suspected of being unhealthy. If a baby cannot adequately take a breath, we must use a syringe to clear the passageway of mucus. A baby needs the power of the throat immediately. Babies, even the youngest ones, are very expressive, whether by crying, screaming, making gurgling noises, or cooing.

In utero, your baby cannot speak or make a sound other than hiccups, but she can hear. Self-expression involves listening, too, so the ears matter a great deal. In fact, the throat center is active very early in fetal development, because we know that babies become familiar with their mother's voice, which has a unique vibratory pattern, while in the womb and prefer it to anyone else's shortly after birth. They even prefer songs or stories heard in utero. Your baby arrives with a clear preference for your voice, your songs, your stories. This means that for your unborn baby, the throat center was operating to receive information through the ears, even if it was muffled somewhat by her watery environment in your belly. The fact that she arrived familiar with your voice vibrations is truly amazing!

Voice is one of the most important early connections that you have to your baby, and each individual voice has a particular vibration. In fact, speech requires that you develop enough control over your breath and your tongue to form different vibrational patterns that convey meaning to a listener. Your baby comes ready to make noises and to cry, but not to speak, because the motor control for the breath and tongue does not yet exist. The throat energetic center must be more energized for this to occur. In the first year of life, you must try to discern what your baby's different sounds mean through their unique vibrational patterns. There are distinct cries for "I am tired," "I am hungry," "I am afraid," and "I am uncomfortable."

Words can be powerful and can be seen in written, spoken, or even musical form. The throat center is involved in every form of creative expression. We must be able to take in information, process it, then give out our own unique expression of it, creating a self-identity as a creative being. A baby takes all that she is from the other seven energy centers and expresses it to others through this center.

Although children learn to form sounds in their first year of life and usually develop words in their second year of life, the throat center typically develops more fully in later childhood, from about six to twelve. During this time she is in school, learning the unique ways in which she can express herself. During these years, your child will have to produce from the throat center in order to create something for her teacher, whether it is spoken, written, drawn, or sung. Depending upon adult reactions, children will become either proud or ashamed of their productions. Those who say "Children should be seen but not heard" are destructively criticizing these children; such criticism can block the throat center. Children who are told lies or who are not encouraged to tell the truth have problems in this area as well.

Many parents complain about crying babies, but a baby's cries have always been music to my ears, because I know the baby is energizing the throat center from which she may one day sing or speak eloquently. Babies are supposed to cry. They cannot speak yet, so it is essential for them to cry to activate the throat center and express themselves. When frustrated parents complain about this, I try to introduce a little humor into the situation by joking that the only thing worse than a whining baby is a parent whining about a whining baby.

When my son was three months old, I put him in a front carrier over my chest and went to the food market to get supplies. The store was noisy, chaotic, and filled with shoppers. My son began to cry unremittingly. I was becoming quite anxious, so I hurried to collect the items I needed and check out. As my son screamed his lungs out, a woman on line in front of me turned and said, "Indian babies never cry." I was not sure what to say, but finally I managed to reply, "I don't have an Indian baby." As we left the store, my son quieted down and became a happy, contented baby once more. My nerves were frayed, but I understood what he had been trying to communicate with his wails, and I tried not to repeat the episode. And contrary to what the woman told me, all babies everywhere do cry at times. They are supposed to cry.

In my career as a therapist, I have dealt a great deal with children who have lost a parent and often have developed a blocked throat center. In one such case, I was introduced to a three-year-old boy who had lost his mother. He came to me as a mute child; although he had been talking articulately before the death of his mother, he had suddenly stopped speaking afterward. Many professionals had tried to determine if it was a physical problem, and he had also been seen by several other therapists. I began by joining him in silence, but playing with him nonverbally in a very animated fashion. Although he tried to block me from his vision, he could not miss the energy of the throat center that I kept sending. He did not speak a word for the first four sessions as we engaged in parallel play. But I knew, because we had bonded, that he could talk and was electively mute due to the emotional trauma he had suffered. I also knew that I could treat him, because after the first session, as he walked out the door acting as though he were unaware of me, he turned back to sneak a look at me, giving himself away. I knew I had him, and I would not let go. In the fifth session, in honor of the fifth energetic center, the throat, he and I hummed a song together for the very first time. That marked the beginning of his recovery period, and we worked together successfully for the next year to open the throat center and talk about the grief of losing a mom. We also had a great deal of fun. As I walked with him, I remembered the old saying "Joy shared is doubled, grief shared is halved." This is true no matter what the trauma suffered.

I have always found it beneficial to unblock the throat center for children and parents. If you bond with your baby early, you will know the magic of the throat center. As your child expresses the pain or joy of a life experience, you will know the healing words to say that make a difference.

The process of bonding expressively with your baby begins by talking softly but animatedly to your baby throughout the day. Her ears need to be stimulated by your vibration, not your loud voice. Your baby's ears are composed of delicate internal structures and need careful handling. Babies favor repetitive, rhythmic sounds. Lullabies are appealing because of their soft, singsong quality. When your baby vocalizes, make eye contact and respond by copying the sounds, to show they have been received and to initiate an energetic throat connection. Act as if a real conversation is taking place. You can say such things as "Is that so?" "Tell me all about it" or "And what else do you want to tell me?" Give your baby time to respond, then answer her vocally. Babies love this and are very excited by the energetic connection. They feel that they have power in the world. They can express themselves and be heard and the world responds. To a baby, you are the world. If you do not respond, the world does not seem like a very friendly place to be.

Physical Purpose

The physical purpose of these exercises is to open up the airways and allow the open flow of energy. When there is a tightening of the throat area, the voice and hence the clear expression of self cannot flow easily and naturally. The genuineness of self-expression shines through only when the throat is relaxed and open.

Psychological Purpose

Encourage your baby's expressions and vocalizations and begin to intuitively understand what she means. This requires the most important parental tool: listening to your baby with the third, or inner, ear. To listen with the third ear is to hear the words and the meanings of the words on more than a literal level. It means to understand the emotion behind the words and the deeper meaning of the words so that you, as a parent, can respond appropriately to the needs expressed.

Yoga Mind

This energetic center is about building bridges. Yoga mind is keenly aware that you are building the bridge of expression from the internal world—the ideas of the mind and the sensations of the body—to the external world. It is important to build strong bridges so that each is connected solidly to the other and so that both sides can be adequately served. The mind cannot exist without being solidly linked to the body, and the body does not operate in a healthy way without the use of the mind. The internal world by itself, unconnected to the external, is a lonely place, and if the external world is never fed with the riches of the internal world, it becomes meaningless. The bridges are vital.

Yoga Technique

The technique for opening up the throat center is very subtle yet highly effective. The stimulation is merely light touch. For the delicate throat center, less is more, and small movements have strong effect. This center includes the ear, which is one of the most sensitive parts of the body, primarily because of the energy meridians located about its perimeter. Therefore, it is essential to modulate your touch so that it is suitable for the baby.

Ritual

Try scenting the room with sage, which can help you speak clearly and feel purified. Operatic music or pieces featuring other beautiful vocals indicate the throat as the great resonator. Decorate the room with soft colors, such as light, silvery blues. Use tulips, daffodils, and hyacinths, which bravely break their way through the wintry ground to herald spring each year. They signify the bravery of speaking the truth clearly from the throat center, no matter how inhospitable the external environment.

Postures for Mom

To get a sense of the resonator of the throat area, put your fingers on either side of your own neck while you hum. You will feel the vibrations. Sing "do, re, mi, fa, so, la, ti, do" to feel the different vibrations and different frequencies of each sound.

CHIN LOCK

1. With your baby lying on the floor in front of you, sit with your legs crossed in a half-lotus position with your hands crossed behind your head and elbows pointing out to the sides.
2. Push your elbows forward and guide your chin down to your chest.
3. Hold for several seconds, then sit up straight while lifting your head and opening your elbows to the sides.
   4. Repeat five times.

EAR PULL

1. With your baby still lying on the floor in front of you, sit in a half-lotus position with your right arm bent over your head so that your right hand touches your left ear.
2. Slide your right hand over your left ear and tip your head to the right.
3. Hold for five to ten seconds.
4. Release your ear and move your head back to the center.
5. Repeat five times.
6. Repeat the exercise five times with your left hand, tipping your head to the left.

UNLOCKING THE JAW

1. While sitting in the half-lotus position with your baby lying on the floor in front of you, consciously relax your entire face. To do so, become aware of the bones and soft tissue in the areas that are often held tightly in order to let them relax. Allow the jaw to release and drop, the mouth to open, the tongue to sit easily in the back of the mouth, the lips to rest naturally (forming no particular expression), the muscles across the chin and cheeks to smooth out, and the forehead to relax all muscle tension. You will feel a sensation of the muscles having "let go."

2. Remain in this state for thirty seconds, or until your baby fusses for more attention.

3. Repeat five times.

Postures for Baby

OUTER EAR MASSAGE

1. Sitting with your legs straight out in front of you, rest your baby faceup on your legs with her head near your ankles.
2. With your index finger, trace the outside of her ears clockwise, starting at the temples, down the face to the lobes, and up around the very outside of the ears.
3. If your baby responds well, repeat two or three times.

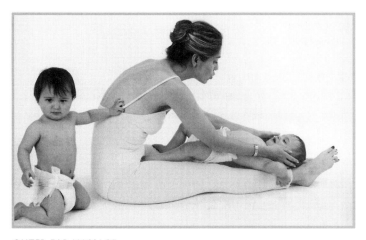

OUTER EAR MASSAGE

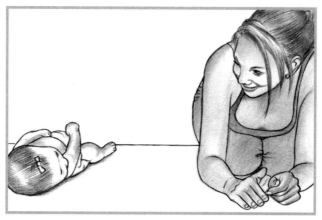

HEAD TWIST TO MOM'S VOICE

HEAD TWIST TO MOM'S VOICE

1. Lay the baby on the floor on her back.
2. Move over to the right side behind the baby's direct vision. Make an inviting noise to attract your baby's attention and to encourage her to look in the direction of your voice.
3. Do the same thing on the left side.
4. Repeat the exercise with two other forms of auditory stimulation— a bell and a rattle are good choices. Always praise your baby for responding.

Postures for Babies Six to Twelve Months

COBRA

1. Place your baby on the floor on her stomach. Kneel behind her with your feet tucked under your buttocks and your toes curled toward the floor.
2. Place both of your hands at your baby's sides.

3. Slide your hands forward under her armpits; continue to slide them forward until your elbows touch the floor and your forearms are up off the floor facing away from you.

4. Turn your palms to face each other and hold your baby's head between them.

5. Rock back toward your heels slightly, keeping your elbows on the floor while lifting the baby's head, arms, and shoulders up off the floor. Her torso should lift a couple of inches while the rest of her body remains on the floor.

6. Pause for a few seconds as your baby gets a chance to look around, then lower her down.

7. Repeat this five times to open up the entire throat and chest area.

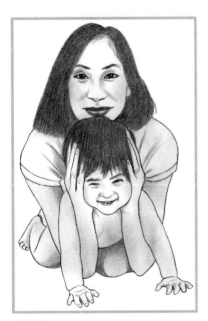

COBRA

Commonly Asked Questions

Q: My baby has a very thick neck; does that mean she will have a powerful throat center?

A: Not necessarily; all babies look a bit like no-necked beings because their necks are not yet strong enough to support the weight of their heads, and consequently the neck is not very clearly defined. Your baby might have a strong throat center, but it is the freedom of her expression and the power of that expression toward others, not the size of her neck, that are evidence of this.

Q: My baby keeps her head turned to the right and resists my turning it to the left. Why?

A: This could be the result of poor sleeping habits and can be corrected by helping the opposite side of the neck develop strength as well. Provide a visual cue to attract the baby's attention to the left. Once she has turned her head, be sure to lengthen the stronger side by stroking the side of the neck to give it a bit of a stretch. Yoga stresses the even development of energy use in the body, so it is important for babies to be able to turn their heads to each side and to lengthen the muscles on either side of the neck, to equalize the neurological patterning and the subtle energy pathways.

Q: My baby cries a lot; should I ignore it?

A: I do not believe in ignoring children or babies when they are expressing themselves. First I ask myself what they are expressing. A baby who cries a lot is unhappy about something. Try to determine whether your baby is tired or hungry, or whether she just needs more time with you. Sometimes the remedy is as simple as letting your baby be close to you, smell you, hear your heartbeat, and feel protected. If your baby does not get enough of that, she may fret a great deal. She is merely expressing a need; it's your job to find out what that need is.

Q: Should I teach my baby to sleep in a noisy environment?

A: No, I do not believe in making certain babies adjust to noise by having them sleep through it. Babies' ears are delicate and in the process of developing. They prefer calmer and softer sounds. They have all their teenage years for loud noises.

For Caregivers

Next to Mom's and Dad's voices, your baby will learn to seek your voice. It will become a symbol for comfort, happiness, and security. So use your voice lovingly, caringly, and liberally so that the baby can fully enjoy and be nurtured by it. Babies do not need discipline; they are too young. They only need love and security, and you are an important part of that process.

Multiple Births

Despite how busy you are, it is very important to spend a little time each day talking to each baby and trying to discern his or her individual, unique nature. Your voice matters, and the vibration of your voice will come to mean a great deal to each of your babies. It also allows you to acquaint yourself with their separate personalities. No matter how similar they may look, they are all different babies with different goals and plans for their lives.

Adopted Babies

Since babies who are adopted do not get the opportunity to hear their adoptive parents' voices before their birth, be sure to provide liberal doses of your voice after the adoption. This sound will come to symbolize you and your relationship with the child. Sometimes babies who have been with a biological mother for some time after birth and then are adopted initially have difficulty making the transition and may be particularly quiet at first. Some adoptive parents fear that it means the baby cannot hear or cannot talk, but usually babies are just making the adjustment to a new set of voices and smells. Patience is the key.

The Head Center

BONDING MENTALLY

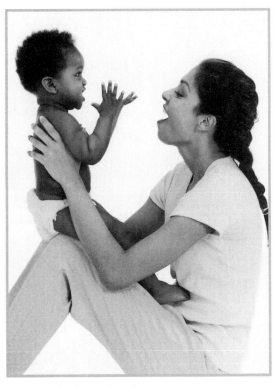

Ariel at six months was very active and loved to be tossed about, preferably upside-down. Her mother was quite concerned, because she perceived Ariel to be a budding tomboy with no intellectual interests. It is amazing how anxious parents are about their baby's behavior and how quick they are to judge it, even at such a young age. She had already been to her pediatrician to ask if Ariel was hyperactive and needed medication to calm down. What an unfortunate step it would have been to medicate this little baby, whose activity was merely a sign that she was developing in the way that was best for her. I have found that in some babies, physical activity stimulates the brain, in particular the vestibular function, in ways that seem to be beneficial to their development. The behavior babies exhibit is often precisely what they need to do in order to develop. We must be

sensitive to their cues and provide what they need. I reassured Ariel's mother and suggested that as long as her daughter was safely supported and not in danger, she should allow Ariel all the stimulation that she desired.

Dreams are the stuff life is made of, and the dreams your baby will have for his life will come from his head center. This chakra is made up of the most advanced part of the brain, the cerebral cortex, where we find abstract and analytic thought and the symbolic language of dreams. As a psychoanalyst trained in dream interpretation, I am able to interpret someone's dreams from this head center to see clearly into the psyche.

The head center, which develops most during the adolescent period, is about the clarity of perception. Related to the upper portion of the head, it includes the eyebrows, forehead, and eyes. The eyes are sometimes described as the windows to the soul. But no matter what the physical eyes see, the head center provides the real truth of perception. The physical eyes alone are not enough to perceive the whole of a situation. For example, one can see someone commit an act, but to see the motivation for the act requires a clear head center. To see clearly and fully the *ajna*, or third eye, as it is sometimes called, is necessary. This is just another way to describe the energetic head center.

The third eye is thought to be in the center of the forehead, above the eyes, but actually it is in perfect alignment with the pituitary gland, which is associated with the head center. The pituitary gland—located behind the center of the forehead and between the eyes several inches inside the brain—is the master gland of the entire body and endocrine system. It is the director of all the hormones that are released and the timing of their release as the body and mind need them for their survival. The pituitary gland is designed to be sure that all functions are as they should be and as your baby needs them. Based upon your perceptions, the head center governs the operation of the whole body and mind. As we psychologists often say, it is perception of reality, not actual reality, that governs behavior. The head center confirms this view.

The head center, with its sensitivity to light through the eyes, acts as the filter through which all thoughts, actions, and desires pass. If the filter is cloudy, then perceptions are distorted, leading to projections and illusions, and actions are muddled. If the filter is crystal clear, then clear perception leads to clear thought and action. Clairvoyance is really just clear perception—seeing clearly without a cloudy filter. This is the goal for all of us and, of course, for your baby.

The head center is also related to wisdom. More than the wisdom of one person, it is the wisdom of the species that is the real focus of the energetic head center. The head center participates in evolutionary development so that the brain knows what evolutionary steps, adjustments, changes, or developments will serve the species best. For example, in the century to come, does humanity need eyes with greater or less sensitivity to light? This question is designed to ensure that the species continues to survive and evolve. Evolution always pushes toward change, no matter the discomfort created, to ensure species survival. The frontal lobes of the cerebral cortex and the pituitary gland are intimately involved in this task. In the head center, species survival more than individual survival is key. That is why our children will continue to evolve and change, even though we cannot yet know what the next decade or century will require of our species. This is the business of the head center.

Your baby has arrived here on Earth with the mental equipment necessary for the challenges to come as well as the challenges that exist right now. Sometimes we parents are a bit behind and our children are a little bit ahead of where things are moving and going. They arrive better prepared for what is coming than we are. We have to work to catch up to them. This is probably the true meaning of the generation gap.

For example, if you are a baby boomer, you arrived on Earth with a brain ready for the sound bytes so popular on television because you grew up in the age of the television. But children today are growing up with the visual byte so necessary for the computer age, as well as a multiple focus for the space age and quick focus, which sometimes is misidentified as short attention span. They arrive ready for MTV and a faster life.

We sometimes call this readiness for what the future brings "higher perception." Just as our computers come installed with the latest versions of operating systems so as to be prepared for the tasks of tomorrow, your baby comes wired for the next evolutionary challenge, which in this case is intergalactic travel. Our little stars are ready to revisit the stars, ready for five-dimensional thought and travel! This is very evident in my private practice. Children five years ago would spend their therapy play time acting as characters from the Indiana Jones movies or other adventure films. But today they play characters who relate to other planets. No one told them to do this; they just have naturally gravitated to the concept of intergalactic travel. This is also the center from which intuition emanates. When synchronizing with your baby, it is the center from which you will intuit your baby's needs.

The brain is the most precious part of the human body. The head center—related to the brain—can be thought of as the master computer or control tower for all your chakras. It can also be described as the leader, the director of the show, for the whole species. The leader of a group is concerned not just with one individual, but rather with the whole group of individuals. A good leader sees farther ahead than the others and directs the group in a visionary way, making plans and thinking of the good of the group, not the good of one. In this way, the head center expands our individual boundaries beyond ourselves to our shared humanity.

The delicate brain floats gently on a water bed of cerebrospinal fluid inside the protective cranial case. There is a pulse to the movement of the fluid surrounding the brain, which skilled osteopaths and craniosacral therapists can sense. But since it is too difficult for most of us to sense, you may or may not feel it as you hold your baby's head delicately between your hands.

Self-reflection and an understanding of how humanity fits into something bigger begin here. The head center operates at a higher vibrational level than the throat center. According to the psychiatrist Carl Jung, the head center is where we find the archetypes and the collective unconscious. An archetype is a universal template, like an architectural plan of the psyche and the identity we have. The fuzzy perceptions of idealized images and despised images of self that block our evolution toward greater wholeness are also found here. The collective unconscious is the memory of the evolution of our species; it is stored in our brains somewhere, to be used as our head center leads us ever forward in our evolutionary path. This shared evolutionary past links us, so we are not alone. It links your baby to all the rest of us and to our ancestors.

At first your baby will not see clearly and definitely the hard, sharp edges of objects, but will have an overall impression of shape, color, and movement. As the eyes mature, they will begin to focus more solidly on the here and now. At first the two sides of babies' brains are largely nondifferentiated, but as it develops, one hemisphere will become dominant, or more dynamic, and the other will become more receptive. Brain hemisphere dominance will eventually show up in a preference for one eye, hand, and foot, but usually not until much later (approximately four to six years). The two eyes will see differently and take in information differently, just as the two legs and two arms will perform differently. Each side of the body will even be formed slightly differently, with one side somewhat larger than the other.

If the permanent center is the originating spark of the artwork that is life, the root center the generator of creative energy, the regenerative center the artist's palette, the solar plexus the decision-making center, the heart center the canvas, and the throat center the creative act, then the head center is the place where the meaning of the artist's painting or creation of the life is understood both by the artist and in terms of the evolution of all artists.

Physical Purpose

In this center, there is a different purpose for the baby than for the adult. For your baby, try to activate the eyes by orienting him and encouraging his visual tracking. For adults, whose eyes have mastered visual tracking, concentrate on developing what I call a "soft focus"—an inner perception, or rather an inner sense, of your baby, whether or not you see him physically.

Psychological Purpose

Your goal is to activate and honor higher perception in your child and to help develop it. Whenever your child shares his or her perceptions, encourage this without judgment.

Yoga Mind

Assume there is nothing wrong with your baby and that he is perfect for what he needs in this life. If he comes with a particular and unusual need, consider this part of his path toward wholeness—not a problem, but part of the process. Expect your baby to have different capabilities than you do. He is supposed to be different because he will be living in a different period of time than you. Resist the temptation to label behavior and seek simple solutions, such as this behavior is normal or deviant. Let the baby and his personality unfold without value judgments.

Yoga Technique

The idea is to work with your child, not against her. You are not adversaries; you are companions on the path of life. As you lead and guide your baby, also allow yourself to learn from your baby. Teaching/learning is a two-way street.

The Ritual

The color most often associated with the head center is indigo, like the midnight blue color seen on the darkest night, when the stars seem to shine most brilliantly. I find this time of night spectacular, because this is the time when dreams occur; with the help of these dreams' profound insight, lives can be reorganized and made anew.

You can try the scent of cloves for memory and clarity or even the scent of chamomile for peace and relaxation. The flower associated with dreams is mimosa. Music should be otherworldly, such as New Age music, since dreams develop from our parallel universe, our dream state, our unconscious.

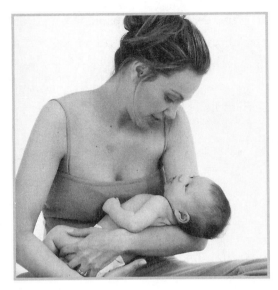

MEDITATIVE POSITION FOR SOFT FOCUS

Postures for Moms

MEDITATIVE POSITION FOR SOFT FOCUS

1. Sit in a half-lotus position and hold your baby in a feeding position. Support your back if it makes you more comfortable.
2. Cradle your baby's head and neck in the crook of your arm.
3. Relax your forehead, close your eyes, and begin to get a sense of your baby through your hands rather than your physical eyes and your vision. As you relax your eyes, your mind will pick up cues about your baby in other ways. We call this inner sense or inner perception.
4. Breathe together with your baby for a few minutes. If you want to listen to music, be sure it supports your meditative mood and feelings, since the head center is about meditative activities.
5. Get a sense of your baby from inside your head. Find a calmness in your mind and quiet your breathing.
6. Hold this posture for one minute or until the baby gets fussy.

Postures for Babies

FOREHEAD MASSAGE

1. With your baby lying vertically on the floor on his back, with his head closest to your ankles, cradle his head in your hands.
2. With your fingers on the sides and back of his neck, place your thumbs at his temples and make circular movements to stimulate the skin.
3. Place your thumbs on top of his forehead and slowly slide them across his forehead down to his ears, as if to smooth out the forehead.
4. Massage the forehead while holding his head steady in your palms and fingers.
5. Continue for one minute or until the baby gets fussy.

EYE TRACKING

This exercise stimulates a baby's ability to track an object visually. Use any red object that attracts your baby's attention, as long as it is not sharp and is big enough for her to see. A good choice would be a red plastic ring, about three to four inches in diameter, suspended by a string.

1. Sit in the half-lotus position and set your baby on the floor facing you and lying on her back.

2. Suspend the ring about eight inches above your baby's eyes and move it from her left side to her right at medium speed to attract her visual attention. If you move the ring too quickly, the baby's eyes will not follow it; if you move it too slowly, the baby will not be interested.

3. Then, still holding the ring above the baby's eyes, move it from the level of her eyes down to her chin and up again.

4. Next, move the ring in a circle. Make the circle slightly bigger than the baby's head. Circle in one direction and then the other to stimulate both eyes.

5. Do each of these movements five times or until your baby becomes tired.

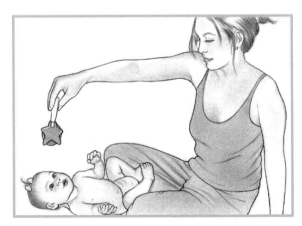

EYE TRACKING

Exercises for Babies Six to Twelve Months

EYE TRACKING

1. With the baby seated in front of you facing out, catch his eye by moving the red ring from side to side.
2. Next move it up and down.
3. Now try moving it circularly to encourage him to use his eyes to track it. You will know he is tracking the object because his head will incline in the direction of the moving object, just as people's heads turn to follow a ball in play in a tennis match.
4. Repeat each movement five times.

Commonly Asked Questions

Q: How can I stimulate my baby's brain and thought process?

A: Different babies receive stimulation in different ways. If you are open to your baby's cues, you will perceive the need and meet it. Don't worry, this happens quite naturally. Remember, all babies need motor, emotional, visual, auditory, and tactile stimulation.

Q: Could my baby be manic-depressive? His moods change so much.

A: Babies' moods do change a great deal. This is completely normal. Be careful not to attach psychiatric labels to a developing baby; let him develop on his own.

Q: Should my baby watch TV while swinging in his swing? Is it bad?

A: I don't think babies can be harmed by watching visual displays, whether on television or in real life, as long as the television is not used as a baby-sitter for extended periods of time. Be sure that your baby is far enough away from the television that the radiation emitted, or the light in the room, does not harm his eyes.

Q: Sometimes my baby averts his gaze from me when I come home from work. Does he recognize me?

A: Of course he recognizes you, but he is registering his anger at your absence during the day. Babies do not have many ways to register such emotions, and they may avert their eyes to indicate displeasure or anger. Give him time, and slowly let him adjust to having you home. He is just sad to have missed you all day.

Q: My baby's eyes seem to focus differently. Is this a problem?

A: This is not an issue of visual acuity. Babies use each eye differently; they have to learn to coordinate their eyes, which adults have already learned. Note how his eyes develop over the next two years. If problems persist, check with your pediatrician or ophthalmologist.

Q: Does this chakra pertain to education?

A: Although this session is about bonding mentally, the chakra does not necessarily involve education. While education is certainly desirable and helpful, it alone does not create a powerful head center. The head center exists in each one of us, whatever our level of schooling.

Multiple Births

Attending to the visual stimulation needs of all your babies can be difficult. It is important to realize that their needs may vary dramatically, so you must assess the differences among them. One may like a great deal of visual stimulation, with much change of color and shape, whereas another may prefer softer, muted colors and slowly changing visual displays. Take note and be sensitive to these needs.

The Crown Center

BONDING BY SPIRITUAL EMPOWERMENT

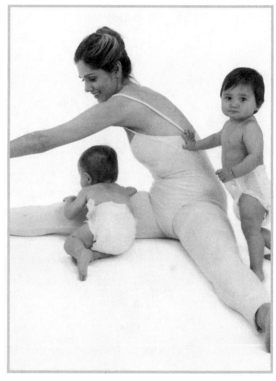

Diana's mother was not sure she believed in the concept of spirit. When we worked on the crown center in Yoga Baby class, she initially felt very uncertain and ill at ease. When I explained that no matter whether she believed in spirit or not, the crown center was about getting in tune with one's own bodily cycles and the cycles of the planet and the universe, she felt more able to accept the crown center as important. I explained that since she struggled with little Diana (6 months) about when to sleep and when to eat, we might try to get their cycles more in tune and Diana more in touch with the day-night cycle. We devised a plan to encourage Diana to sleep for greater stretches during the night and to stay awake for longer periods of time during the day. This suited her mother very well. She began to understand that these cycles were related to the activation of the crown center.

Just as every pool of water on Earth reflects the Moon, every baby reflects the entire universe. The energetic crown center, at the very top of the head, is considered the spiritual or meditative center—the part of us that is in touch with the universe. For this reason, the activities of this center, which develops most prominently during early adulthood, include meditative techniques. If you placed a tiny round bowl right over the top of the baby's head, you would have traced the perimeter of the crown center. It is defined by the larger of the two soft spots your baby arrives with; these two areas are the fontanels, where the bones of the skull have not yet fused and only a protective membrane separates the delicate brain from the outside world. Hard bone has not yet developed to close the crown center— your baby arrives open to the heavens. She must live here several months to become grounded on Earth, and during this time the fontanels gradually close and the baby forgets where she comes from.

The pineal gland is associated with the spiritual center. The gland is sensitive to light and is responsible for the precise adjustments of the autonomic nervous system and endocrine system that are part of our sleep-wake cycle and which are so necessary for health. Melatonin is the hormone produced by this gland. Melatonin regulates sleep cycles and helps coordinate the body's biological functions with the external environment. It can be used to reset one's biological clock when it is thrown off by jet lag. The pineal gland directs all the body systems to prepare for behavior, while awake or asleep.

We know that exposure to full-spectrum light is essential for health and that artificial lighting, especially fluorescent lighting, is not beneficial to health. When there is insufficient exposure to full-spectrum light, we run the risk of depression, chronic fatigue, and higher levels of stress hormones. In children a lack of sufficient light has been associated with hyperactivity, learning disorders, and visual difficulties. Seasonal affective disorder, or SAD, is a depressive condition associated with the winter months, when full-spectrum light is minimal.

Over a hundred bodily functions have been correlated with the diurnal cycle. When we alter this rhythm with artificial lighting, jet lag, or irregular hours, we throw off the body's central coordination and natural rhythms. This does not mean that we must make our babies adhere to rigid schedules. For example, working parents can extend their baby's day until much later at night so they can spend time with her before bedtime, as long as they make sure their baby gets enough sleep. Babies can definitely adjust their bodies to this, and it is by far more desirable for a baby to see her parents than to go to sleep according to a predetermined schedule.

Although most would say that the product of the crown center is melatonin, I would say the very best products of the crown center are daytime and nighttime dreams. They are our key to what goes on with us during the night. If not for dreams, what would we know of our nighttime experiences?

Every being needs both waking and sleeping time. Sleep brings healthy REM periods, when dreams are made—dreams unique to the dreamer, just as each person's daytime life has its own unique quality and experiences.

Although we interpret dreams through the head center, the dreams themselves come through the crown center. This is the place of inspiration, where new ideas come to us unbidden, like a bolt of lightning—and for many people this is in the guise of dreams during sleep. We know that babies dream. If you watch your little one sleep, you will see her face change—she will suck, smile, laugh, and become animated, all in the midst of sleep. What is she seeing? We know only that she is in the midst of REM sleep, which is when dreams occur.

Just as every day must have its night, the crown center ties us and our bodies to the cycles of life. The pineal gland has sometimes been called the seat of the soul, the home of the inflow of universal spiritual energy; it is your baby's connection to the Higher. No matter what your conception of a higher force—whether you call it God, Yaweh, the One, Brahman, the All, the Universe, the Light, or just Higher Energy—the crown center is its earthly home. One can be unaware of it, ignore it, denounce it, or decide it does not exist, but I believe it is always there, just like the galaxy, waiting to be seen. Some people never look up at the stars, but the stars are still there always shining. This crown center is the spot from which the halo for saints emanates. It is the same spot from which Buddha's flame is glowing atop his head. It is the place where the crown is placed for the symbol of highest earthly power and authority. It is the Highest.

The story I like best about the crown center is an Indian fable in which God is discussing where to hide man's ultimate powerhouse, his soul, so that no one can steal it and abuse another with its power. He considers placing it atop the highest mountain, deep within a cave, or at the bottom of the ocean, but finally he decides against these because it will be too easy for man to find and steal the soul. Finally, he decides to hide the soul deep within man because man will never think to look there and it will be safe for all time.

The crown center is the soul's hiding place. The crown center brings with it all the power that any man can ever want—to be in union with the universe, to be in rhythm with the night and the day and the cycle of the seasons.

If the permanent center is the originating spark of the artwork that is life, the root center the generator of creative energy, the regenerative center the artist's palette, the solar plexus the decision-making center, the heart center the canvas, the throat center the creative act, and the head center the place where the artist's creative meaning is understood, then the crown center is the place of inspiration and light that guides the artist throughout the creation of life.

In psychology we call the crown center the transpersonal self, for it expands far beyond self, beyond even humanity. It expands your baby beyond himself, beyond his family, beyond his species and into the Heavens, into the solar system and the galaxy from which he came. How your baby maintains his connection with the universe will depend on his life experiences and on you and your attitudes toward the Higher.

What is unity consciousness? Think of it as the way we are all connected, so that what happens to one affects all of us. As scientists have proven, the flutter of something as small as a butterfly's wings on the other side of the world may be felt as the whisper of a breeze upon your cheek on a summer night on this side of the world. Think of how a drop of water from the ocean is changed to vapor, which rises to form clouds, which then flows down on the Earth as rain, is gathered and drunk by you, is transformed into the liquid of a cell in your body, and finally is returned to the Earth upon your death, to continue its journey ever onward. That drop of water you drink has been here, constantly recycled and recycled and transformed, for billions of years since the Big Bang. We are all connected.

The effect of a closed crown center is probably best seen in divisive religious beliefs, in which one group feels they are the only ones who have the spiritual way and that all the other groups are wrong. A closed crown center results in rigidity of thought about spiritual matters and a feeling of wrong versus right. This is not the nature of an open crown center. Your baby arrives with her very own soul, her very own share of infinity right there in the top of her head. In the Yoga Baby program we stimulate and honor it.

What your baby will say, decide, or ask about the world will be her own unique view of the world and how she fits into it. It is important to treat these discussions seriously and allow for her thoughts. When children perceive a bigger worldview, one that gives meaning and purpose to the world and explains how they fit into it, there is hope. These children spontaneously exhibit the Golden Rule, because it flows naturally from their perception of how they fit into a bigger scheme. This is the pure gold of a clear, powerful crown center—unity consciousness.

Physical Purpose

Concentrate on stimulating the brain so that the sleep-wake cycles are adjusted to the cycles of the planet as the Earth turns on its axis and revolves around the sun and as our galaxy spins in the universe. We are all affected by the changes inherent in these cycles, and we need to make physical adjustments to stay in tune with the cycles. The change of seasons is the most obvious way in which people adjust their lives. Not only do we dress differently, but we also alter our diet and exercise patterns based upon seasonal changes.

Psychological Purpose

Try to be aware of your connection and your baby's connection to the universe, to participate in unity consciousness and feel a part of *all*. This is a way to get in touch with your baby's spirituality.

Yoga Mind

We are all part of the cosmos, and when we are in touch with that connection and feel part of it, we enter unity consciousness.

Yoga Technique

The objective of the crown center is to give value to a baby's daytime and nighttime activities, because both are necessary for a baby's health.

The Ritual

Use neroli flowers, which encourage joy and uplifting. Frankincense, for spirituality and meditation, and citrus oils, for revitalization, are other ideal scents to use during your crown center session. The color that best represents the crown center is violet, but personally I prefer gold, like the gold of a crown. I always picture diamonds in the crown because of the pure clarity of the stones, like shining stars in the sky. I love to use harp music during the following exercises, though the sitar is considered a sacred instrument and sitar music is thought of as a pathway to the Highest. Choose whatever music you associate with the sacred.

Postures for Mom

CHILD'S POSE ON HEAD

1. With your baby lying on her back on the floor, about two or three feet in front of you, sit back on your heels with your knees folded.
2. Drop your head forward till the top of your head is aimed toward the floor.
3. Let your arms and hands hang at your sides with the backs of your hands resting on the floor and your palms facing up. Try to let your head droop lower than your heart.

4. Hang the crown of your head as close to the floor as you can so that you are slightly resting the top of your head on the floor. Observe the effect of this exercise on your body. Because all three centers in the head and their glands are stimulated, you will notice a light-headed feeling—a visual dizziness accompanied by a thick feeling in the throat area that makes speech more difficult.

Postures for Baby

SENSE THE FONTANELS

1. Sitting back on your heels with the baby cradled in your arms in the feeding position, rest two fingers of one hand lightly on the top of your baby's head (the larger fontanel, or soft spot) and feel her pulse.
2. Hold for about thirty seconds.
3. Notice the quality of the pulse and condition of the membrane that covers the spot. The pulse is regular and easily determined, though not extremely strong. The membrane is taut, neither sunken nor protruding. This is a perfect spot to get a general feeling for your baby's overall well-being. Depending upon how well or sick your baby feels, there will be a discernible difference in the top of the head and the pulse felt. Take note of what the fontanel feels like in a healthy state.

HEADSTAND PREP

1. Sit with your legs together and extended out in front of you.
2. Place your baby on top of your legs on her back with her head touching the tops of your feet. Hold the baby securely.
3. Relax the backs of your knees as you gently bend them. Support the

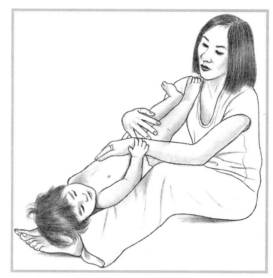

HEADSTAND PREP

baby firmly. The baby's head lowers as the knees lift.

4. Let the baby's head rest between your ankles and feet. Hold for a few seconds only.

5. Now return your legs to the straight starting position, the baby held in between them.

6. Repeat the movement five times.

HEAD SPIRAL

1. Sitting V-legged or on your knees, cradle the baby in your left arm as if you were going to feed him.

2. Place your right hand on top of his head and feel the heat.

3. Take two fingers and trace the direction of the spiral of the hair on the top of the head, keeping your touch extremely light. This is not a massage; it is a gentle touch of the crown center.

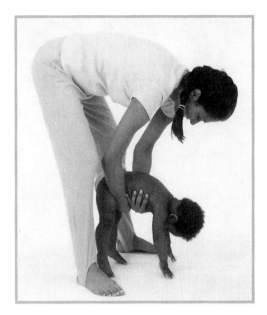

DOWNWARD DOG

Postures for Babies Six to Twelve Months

DOWNWARD DOG

1. Stand and have your baby stand up in front of you, facing out.
2. Hold your right hand around your baby's middle.
3. Place your left hand behind the baby's head.
4. Bend forward and urge your baby to tip forward at the same time and touch his head or hands to the floor. You may wish to move your left hand to the baby's chest and belly to support the upper body while he is in this position.
5. Hold a few seconds, then return to the standing position.
6. Do this five times.
7. Do not your push your baby's head down, but rather let your body lead the movement by tipping over. Be sure to applaud all attempts; this position takes time and patience.

Commonly Asked Questions

Q: I'm afraid of upside-down poses. Can they hurt my baby?

A: We do only a preparation for a headstand, which is a very gentle way to stimulate the blood flow to the brain, and we hold the position for only a few seconds. This is done slowly and carefully. If you follow these instructions and maintain the position briefly, it will not harm your baby. However, babies should not remain upside-down for more than a few seconds.

Q: When do the fontanels close?

A: The bone hardens gradually over the first five to six months of life for the fontanel at the back of the head and at the first year for the fontanel at the top of the head. The size of the fontanels varies from 1 to 3 inches.

Q: How can I tell whether the pulse in the top of my baby's head is healthy or unhealthy?

A: Any deviation from the pulse normally felt in the top of the head means the baby should be checked out. The most common sign of ill health, however, is the fontanel. If it is sunken, the baby could be dehydrated. If it is bulging out, the baby may have an infection. In either case, call your child's pediatrician immediately.

Q: How do I know if my baby will be very spiritual?

A: Everyone is a spiritual being with a connection to the Higher. Your baby's ability to connect to the Higher is a lifetime journey nurtured by the relationship bond with parents through unconditional love.

Q: Is the crown center connected to religion?

A: Although the crown center is associated with spirituality, it is not equated with religion. Religion is man's interpretation and sometimes misinterpretation of the spiritual. According to Carl Jung, "religion is man's greatest block to spirituality"—which suggests we often misinterpret our spiritual connection. The crown center is not about right and wrong. Those are man's issues.

Q: I don't believe in spirit, so why should the crown center matter to me?

A: The crown center is about connecting to the cycles of life and the cycles of the universe, and that refers to connecting with nature. It is not necessary to believe in God or to believe in spirit or spiritualism to recognize this connection.

Adopted Babies

Your baby may come to you with a biorhythm different from yours, because of her experience in utero with a different biological mother. Therefore, you may have to adjust to each other's biological clock until you get more synchronized. Sometimes, we talk about "morning people" and "night owls," but what we are really talking about are their biorhythms. Please remember to be sensitive to this and not critical of the differences as you make the adjustment to each other.

Multiple Births

Different babies have different personalities and can even have slightly different sleep-wake cycles and different sleep needs. Please remember to adjust your schedules and plans according to the individual needs of the babies. One baby may need to be put down first consistently because she tends to need to sleep earlier. There's no need to feel that you are slighting one baby by always putting the same one down first. The important part is to respect each one's individual sleep needs.

Observing Temperament in Baby and Mom

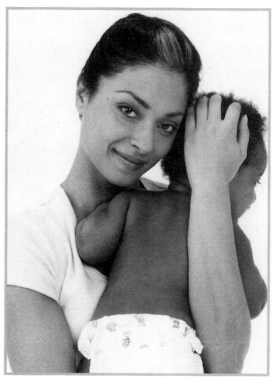

Temperamental differences between parent and baby can make bonding with your baby a challenge. Fortunately, the Yoga Baby program is designed to help bridge such gaps.

Psychologists have observed that babies have their own individual natures from birth. Sometimes these are called temperament; others call them personality. In my research in psychology, I gave psychological tests to hundreds of babies within their first month of life and then retested them every six months for the next several years.

What I found amazing was how individual differences among those babies were quite obvious at just a few days or weeks of age. These differences turned out to be rather stable over time. The other psychologists and myself would play a game of seeing if we could match the original personality descriptions of one-month-old babies with the two- and three-year-old children returning to the center for reevaluation. We were quite accurate in matching the early personality profiles with the older children, suggesting that these little stars arrive with personalities of their own.

Temperament is the behavioral style of a baby or child, the way in which he behaves, and his individual pattern of reacting to the outside world and the people in it. In 1937 Freud acknowledged that "each individual ego is endowed from the beginning with its own peculiar dispositions and tendencies." The concept of temperament in children was reintroduced and researched extensively by Alexander Thomas, Stella Chess, and Herbert Birch in their classic New York Longitudinal Study (NYLS) on temperament in children in 1963. Based on their original research, numerous psychological tests have been devised for observing infants and children, with the hope of bringing some order to our observations of individual differences. According to these psychologists, there are nine categories of reactivity that make up the composite temperament profile for your baby. The categories include: activity level, rhythmicity, approachability, adaptability, intensity, threshold of response, mood, distractibility, attention span, and persistence. I have added a tenth category, soothability, which is related to emotional intelligence.

Activity Level

One of the first indications of your baby's temperament is how active he is. What's the level, tempo, and frequency of his activity? Keep in mind that the activity levels for different age groups look different. An active two-month-old has physical limitations that an active one-year-old does not have. Is your baby in motion much of the time? Is he moving while you perform the basic daily chores of feeding, dressing, diapering, and bathing him, or is he quiet? Is he in the same place you left him in the playpen when you return to the room? Observe your baby over the course of several days and average his activity levels—does he fall closer to the low or high end of the activity scale?

Rhythmicity

Rhythmicity is the degree of regularity of your baby's repetitive biological functions. How regular and predictable are his basic physical activities, such as waking and sleeping, eating, and bowel and bladder functions? Some babies are very rhythmic and eat, sleep, and defecate at predictable times, but others are minimally rhythmic—or arrhythmic— and hence very unpredictable, changing even from day to day. Such babies do not go to sleep, wake up, nap, or get hungry at about the same time every day. As a result, their bowel and bladder functions do not usually happen with regularity, either. Therefore these babies may seem somewhat unpredictable, and it becomes difficult to anticipate how each day can be planned and organized.

Approachability

What is your baby's initial reaction to new situations, new people, new procedures, new toys, new places? Does he approach them or avoid them? Some babies love everything novel, actively seeking out things that are exciting and new, while others react negatively to anything new and different and tend to withdraw. The test is to see how long it takes your baby to warm up to and grab something new. If it takes more than five minutes to attract his attention, it means he warms up slowly to this new item. If he shows visual interest during the five-minute interval, he is not withdrawing but is visually exploring the stimuli and therefore approaching it.

Adaptability

How quickly does your baby adapt or adjust to something new and return to a calm state? Adaptability is a lifelong skill we all need to cultivate, but some babies are born more able to adapt than others. This can be determined by how quickly your baby adapts his behavior to a change in routine, such as when new foods or new clothing is introduced that may call for a different set of behaviors than he has previously shown.

Intensity

How intense are your baby's emotional reactions? Some babies come across as very dramatic, often displaying intense reactions. Other babies are remarkably mild in their reactions, even to seemingly alarming situations. A mild reaction would be a physical wince, but not a loud cry, to a strong stimulus, such as a diaper pin prick. A strong reaction would be a wailing cry over something rather simple, such as the mother adjusting the baby's clothing slightly.

Threshold of Response

Babies have different thresholds of response to stimulation. How much stimulation do you need to give your baby to get a response? Some parents say, "You can do anything to him, it won't bother him." Others say, "He is so sensitive, he is aware of the smallest shift in his blanket at night and wakes up." Some babies are remarkably keen at noticing even the slightest change in their food. Even if you try to introduce a hint of fruit in the cereal, they sense it and refuse it. Others would eat anything without response no matter how saturated the food is with new ingredients.

Mood

What is your baby's mood like for most of the day—pleasant, joyful, and happy, or unpleasant, unfriendly, and unhappy? Babies' moods may also vary a great deal throughout the day, so look for the predominant mood that your baby displays. Usually parents will agree about whether the predominant mood is a positive one or a negative one.

Distractibility

How distractible is your baby? If your baby encounters a new stimulus while he is involved in a physical activity, does he persist at the original activity or drop it and pick up the distraction? If your baby is feeding and the telephone or doorbell rings, does he stop feeding for several seconds? If the baby tends to continue what he was doing, without interruption, he can be considered less distractible.

Attention Span

Babies also vary in attention span. Attention span is judged by the length of time your baby pursues a particular activity. Generally, babies have rather brief periods of attention. Usually a minute or two is a good sign of a strong attention span in the first three months of life.

Persistence

Persistence is the baby's ability to maintain an activity in spite of obstacles, such as continuing to crawl toward a desired goal despite impediments like small toys or other objects placed in his pathway. As another example, does he continue visually exploring his crib mobile even when other things are happening in the room? In other words, does he persist in a goal even when frustrated?

Soothability

Soothability refers to how easily a baby can be soothed or can soothe himself and is related to the baby's development of emotional intelligence. It is an absolutely essential skill for the emotional development of children. Some babies can be readily soothed after being upset, while others can seem inconsolable no matter what you do to calm them.

Psychological tests that are designed to rate a baby's temperament objectively compare your child's responses to those of hundreds of babies at specific ages across all categories. To give you an informal and subjective look at your baby's temperament, we suggest that you, your spouse, and your caregiver fill out the questionnaire that follows for both your baby and yourselves.

According to common belief, the greater the similarity between your scores, the stronger the match and the more manageable you will find your baby. The greater the differences between you and your baby's scores, the more you will perceive the baby as unmanageable. From my viewpoint, however, the greater the differences, the greater the challenge in bridging this temperamental gap to be more in tune with your baby. As a therapist, I am always intrigued by challenges. Besides, temperament is not unchangeable, and it is absolutely affected by your parenting style and the environment. Even if your baby has a difficult temperament, it can be modified through your keen awareness and your willingness to be more in tune with him.

From a psychological perspective, the more energy required from parents to bridge the temperament gap with their baby, the more they will feel enriched by their efforts. Challenges imply learning. Although it takes more energy and patience to bond with a baby who is temperamentally very different from you, there can be an even sweeter joy in the close bond that results.

BABIES WITH A HIGH SCORE

Babies who have a high Total Manageability Score are likely to be rather predictable in their daily routines, with a strong ability to adapt to whatever unexpected turn of events might occur. They can be very persistent, with a good attention span when motivated toward a goal. Their moods tend to be upbeat, but if there are instances when they are upset, they can be easily soothed. Some would consider such children to be "easy" babies, but this depends upon the parent and his or her temperament level. Since this baby may tend to be curious and intellectually demanding, it is important to keep him stimulated.

Let's look at Barry, a baby who has a high Total Manageability Score. He is average in activity level and quite agreeable to whatever happens. He desires what is new and different, and always is alert for what-

TEMPERAMENT OBSERVATION SCALE*

Directions: Please rate your baby in the following eleven categories from Low to Medium to High to indicate the level of each you have observed. Circle your choices, then have each parent and caregiver fill out a separate questionnaire about themselves.

Score	1	2	3
Activity level	High	Med.	Low
Rhythmicity	Low	Med.	High
Approachability	Low	Med.	High
Adaptability	Low	Med.	High
Intensity	High	Med.	Low
Threshold of response	Low	Med.	High
Mood	Low	Med.	High
Distractibility	High	Med.	Low
Attention span	Low	Med.	High
Persistence	Low	Med.	High
Soothability	Low	Med.	High

A modified version of a Sample Observation Scale of Temperament from the Chess, Birch, and Thomas original version.

Mother's score: _____

Father's score: _____

Caregiver's score: _____

Baby's score: _____

Add all the scores for a Total Manageability Score:

High scores: 26 to 33

Medium scores: 19 to 22

Low scores: 11 to 18

ever is going to happen next. Things cannot be too lively for him. He likes being around a large family and watching them all interact. He does not like to be totally on his own unless he has new toys to play with.

Barry's mother finds his need for a continual stream of new stimulation exhausting, yet he is a very agreeable baby. She scored in the average range, but low on the approachability category. She likes routine and sameness, and this was the sticking point between the two. I had to help her realize that if she provided the baby with novel stimulation each day, or allowed him to find it safely for himself, she would have an agreeable baby. If she did not provide for this need, then her own need for routine would be disrupted by a very unhappy baby. She could give him adequate stimulation by making each day's activities new and different—varying the toys presented, the activities engaged in, the destinations planned for outings, and the people he sees each day. However, the basic structure for the day could remain the same to suit the mother's need for routine.

BABIES WITH A MEDIUM SCORE

If your baby scored in the medium range, she is likely to be an agreeable baby on the surface but not especially predictable in her schedule. She has an average activity level, and may require a bit more stimulation to get a reaction. She tends to approach and withdraw from the novel in equal amounts. If upset, she may be able to soothe herself at times, but not at others. This baby requires work because in each category she can exhibit some of the extremes. The trick is knowing which response she exhibits at which time and how to work with it.

Sally is a perfect example of this profile. She is fairly adaptable half the time but not the other half. Her mother finds it difficult to determine how she will react at any given time, and why. Sally persists at a goal until she seemingly has had enough and then she loses interest altogether. Her mother has a hard time convincing her to keep up with any task. Sally's mood is neutral and she does not have many highs or lows; this upsets her mother, who is rather intense in all her reactions.

Sally's mother scored in the low range, with high intensity, high activity, high distractibility, and low persistence. This gap between mom and baby was difficult to bridge. Her mother needed greater understanding in order to be able to figure out how Sally was likely to react, and why. To simplify matters, we picked one category to focus on: mood. Mother had to learn to accept Sally's neutral mood as different from hers and take it as a sign that Sally was all right. This made her less demanding of Sally, and Sally felt more at ease.

BABIES WITH A LOW SCORE

If your baby's score is low, he is likely to be hard to soothe when upset, and his mood may often seem negative. Some parents find this troubling. If his attention span is short and his persistence low, you may have a hard time motivating him toward a goal. If he is also slow to adapt to new situations, you may find you need to stick to a regular schedule to keep his mood neutral. If his activity level is low, it may be easier because he will be less demanding. But if his activity level is high, you have the challenging task of keeping him on as even a keel as you can. You may find yourself feeling slightly unbalanced.

An example of a low-scoring baby is Norman, whose mom found his temperament very difficult because she is rhythmic and somewhat placid. She scored mainly in the average range of all categories, and she considered Norman a handful. To help the two synchronize their schedules, I suggested that his mother be less rigid with her routine and simultaneously try to keep Norman's daily activities a bit more regular, in the hope that somewhere in the middle they could meet and make a match.

SIMILAR PARENT AND BABY TEMPERAMENTS

It is true that the more similar the temperament between parent and baby, the "easier" the parent perceives the baby to be. One of our moms and her baby son Julian were so similar, their faces even looked exactly alike. They could have practically burped at the same time. We used to laugh about the fact that they resembled two peas in a pod and asked if they were sure they weren't really twins born thirty years apart.

OPPOSITE PARENT AND BABY TEMPERAMENTS

The more different the temperament between baby and parent, the more "difficult" the parent may perceive the baby to be. Ursula and her mom are a good example. Ursula is a rather placid baby who is agreeable to whatever happens—changes in routine, activity, situation, and people don't bother her much. She is not especially reactive or intense. Her mother is very intense and it takes very little to get a reaction from her. Ursula's mother scored low on several key temperament categories: intensity, mood, and threshold. She was convinced that her baby's inactivity was the result of some intellectual inferiority that she was determined to stimulate her out of. So by the age of six months she had enrolled her in every program one could imagine. This was particularly upsetting to little Ursula, whose preference was to do a few things slowly. But her mother would not leave her alone. It was very difficult to convince her that with Ursula, less was more and that she was lucky she had a baby so different from herself, as ultimately this would make the match very positive. If Ursula and her mother had both been highly reactive, they could have been a better match initially, but as Ursula grew, highly volatile situations would have been difficult to avoid. With time and patience, Ursula's mother adjusted her reactivity, and this gave Ursula some much-needed relief.

Arrhythmic Babies and Parents

If your baby is arrhythmic, has intense reactions, a low threshold of response, and a low soothability score, this means more work for you as parents. You are likely to be tired because of his erratic sleep schedule and frustrated by his inability to soothe himself. This baby will prove very difficult for a rhythmic parent. If, however, you are arrhythmic and your baby is too, you will find this less concerning than the average parent.

Remember, the parent that is more similar to his or her baby will have an easier time with the baby. Their rhythms and temperaments are more in sync naturally. But no matter the difference between a parent and baby, a motivated parent with understanding can create synchronization.

How does knowledge of temperament help in the Yoga Baby program? Understanding your child's temperament is the beginning of understanding his unique nature. It is essential to understand who each of you is and what your similarities and differences are. Where differences exist, it is important to understand how to bridge the gaps so that a deep bond can form. The more you know, the deeper the enhancement of your experience with the Yoga Baby program.

Continuing Yoga Baby with the Mobile Baby

(TWELVE TO TWENTY-FOUR MONTHS)

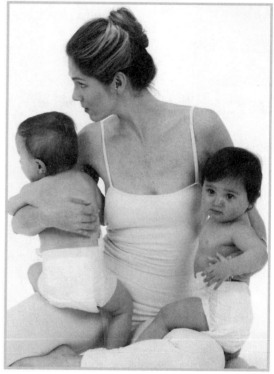

Congratulations! This is the year your baby will start walking and talking. The first time your baby is able to get out of his crib without your assistance, you'll realize that you have a full-fledged one-year-old on your hands.

Your older baby can continue to benefit from yoga. Because the bond you create with your baby is lifelong and always changing, it is important to remember that the Yoga Baby program is a start to a process that will continue to unfold. Each stage of child development leads to the next parental dilemma and adjustment. It takes a continual flow of learning to get in rhythm with your baby, and each age brings new challenges. Yoga, too, is a lifelong practice, and it can help you meet these challenges.

Now that your baby is one year old, he has made enormous strides in his development. He is prepared to physically explore everything he can get his hands on. He has become a small person of boundless energy, because all his energetic centers are activated. He explores everything and moves about ceaselessly all day until he finally collapses into sleep at night. He may even resist sleep, because he feels life is too exciting to miss a moment. Because your child is so focused on movement, you'll need to modify your postures to accommodate a moving baby. Similarly, you'll learn to take your quiet moments as your baby allows them. Meditative time is brief.

Postures are never forced upon a baby; rather, a baby is encouraged and coaxed into certain movements and then rewarded. Expect to use your psychological skills to motivate your baby, and be sure to make it all fun. I provide lots of positive feedback with praise and applause. I also use props when needed, because as babies are learning to walk, they need equipment or furniture that is solid and can support their weight as they lean against it.

You can use more verbal cues now, as your baby's language develops, to help initiate movements or encourage her to get into certain poses. For example, if you need to get your baby's feet to her head, try saying "Kiss your feet" or "Smell your feet." For forward poses, give the cue "Go to sleep," or try any phrase that your baby responds to that helps her initiate the movement. You can even develop your own labels for these movements that will become familiar to your baby. For example, try calling the Cobra position the "Snake," and encourage your baby to lean her head back while making the hissing sounds of a snake. Don't hesitate to be creative with the following postures.

The Root Center

The purpose of the movements in the root center is to connect solidly to the Earth so that as the baby begins to walk, he is well balanced and his spine is perfectly aligned.

In the root center, we focus on all the prerequisite movements necessary for your baby to crawl and walk forward and backward, as well as stand erect with his weight evenly distributed. In order to drive energy into your baby's legs and feet, begin by encouraging crawling movements.

CRAWLING

1. Sit on your heels on the floor and set your baby on the floor in front of you in a sitting position facing outward.
2. Help him shift toward the right so that his weight is on his right hip with his legs slightly extended to the left side.
3. Urge him to lean his weight on his hands, which he can set on the floor in front of him while keeping his arms outstretched for support.
4. Gently move his right leg back behind him, aligning the left leg with it so he is resting on all fours (two hands, two knees). If he retreats back to the floor, leave him in this position for a few moments, but then gently move him back to the crawl position.
5. Place a toy a short distance away from him on the floor and help move his right hand forward, then left knee forward, then left hand forward, then right knee forward, and so on until he is within reaching distance of the toy. If he retreats to sitting on one hip and crawling with only one leg, he is still progressing. This is a wonderful introduction to crawling.

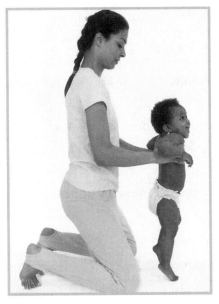

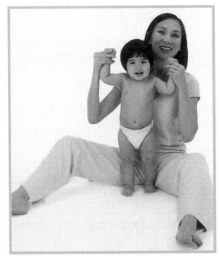

STANDING

WALKING

STANDING

1. Kneel on the floor with your baby lying on his back on the floor in front of you. His head should be closer to your body, with his feet extended out.
2. Hold his hands firmly within your own and help him pull up to a sitting position; then release back down.
3. Practice this move five times. This will help build essential walking muscles in the abdomen.
4. Next, help him pull himself up from a sitting to a standing position. After he stands for a few moments with full support (hold him around his torso under the armpits), help him back down to a sitting position.
5. Do this exercise together five times daily until he has the strength to stand up for several minutes.
6. Once he is able to stand erect, transfer his support from your hands

to a solid piece of furniture. It will take a great leap of faith on his part to let go of you and trust that you have given him suitable support, so he may need loving encouragement in order to let go of your hands. After he has let go, allow him to support himself for a few minutes before resuming your hand support.

7. Repeat this for several days and weeks, if necessary, until he demonstrates the strength and willingness to take his first step.

Some babies are eager to take their first steps, while others are very hesitant. In reaching this milestone, you may support your baby's body under his arms or around his middle. When he develops more upper-body strength, transfer your support to his pelvic area so that his upper body is free to move independently and twist from side to side. Also, let him jump up and down as much as he likes while you hold him in order to stimulate contact between solid ground and his own two feet.

WALKING

1. In order to encourage your baby to walk, hold his hands and allow him to take steps while you either sit or kneel on the floor or stand behind him.

2. Grasp his hands in yours to steady his body as he learns the feel of movement.

3. Be sure to move his left hand forward as his right foot moves forward and his right hand forward as his left foot moves forward; this will help him maintain balance.

4. Your baby will want more aid in walking than you will be able to provide, so be sure to have toys that will stimulate him. Toys that must be pushed to produce music and little red wagons are excellent stimuli for this purpose. Be sure they are at the proper height for your baby to stand and walk with.

The Regenerative Center

The purpose of the exercises for the regenerative center is to open up the sacrum for ease of movement from the hip area. This will allow your child to twist, turn, and walk with ease.

AB WORK

1. Place your baby flat on his back on the floor, feet toward you. Sit at his side.
2. With one hand, gently take hold of the baby's legs behind the knees. With the other hand, support the back of the baby's neck while lifting the torso and legs up to position the body in the shape of a V.
3. Hold this posture for several seconds, then gently release both your baby's torso and legs down to the floor at the same time.
4. Repeat this position five times to help your baby develop his abdominal muscles.

KISS FEET

1. While sitting in a V-legged position, lay your baby on his back on the floor in front of you and guide his feet up to his mouth to "kiss."
2. Hold a few seconds, then release down.
3. Repeat five times.

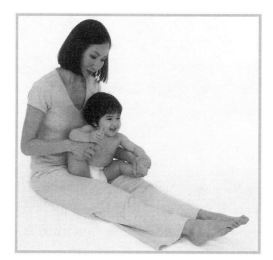

PEDALING

PEDALING

1. Sit in a V-legged position with your baby lying flat on the floor with his head away from you, or sitting up in front of you on your straight, extended legs, facing outward.
2. Help him pedal his feet with bent knees in a forward direction, then reverse for several repetitions. Learning to bring the knee into the chest while pedaling is particularly helpful for later exercises.

The Solar Plexus Center

The purpose of movements in this center is to provide a strong center of gravity with greater flexibility in the spine. This will allow your baby to freely perform twisting movements.

STANDING FORWARD BEND

1. Stand up while your baby stands in front of you facing outward.
2. Anchor your baby's feet by placing your bare feet on top of his so that he is solidly connected to the ground to counterbalance the weight movement forward.
3. While holding your baby at the waist, bend him forward, keeping his knees as straight as possible. Try to avoid letting his knees collapse to the floor.
4. Once he gets the hang of it, let him bend over for several seconds, then return to a standing position.
5. Let him rest for a few seconds before repeating the movement. Do this five times.

YOGIC SLEEP

1. Sit in a V-legged position with your baby lying flat on the floor horizontally in front of you, with his head pointed toward one of your inner thighs and his feet toward the other.
2. Lift his feet to his nose while lifting the back of his head up to meet his feet at the center of his body.
3. Hold for ten seconds, release, then repeat five times. Be sure to allow the baby to move about the room freely between repetitions.

The Heart Center

The purpose of movements for the heart area is to open the chest cavity for the heart to pump the life force through the body and give the lungs more space for easier breathing.

FULL BOW POSE

1. Sit on the floor in a V-legged position with your baby horizontally in front of you as he lies on his stomach.
2. Reach underneath his legs and lift them with bent knees so that his upper thighs are off the floor.
3. At the same time, with the baby's arms along his sides, lift his head and chest up from the floor. If your baby has a good degree of flexibility, grasp his two hands behind his back in one of your hands and his two feet in your other hand and have them meet behind his back in the center of the torso. If your baby lacks flexibility, simply lift the legs and head up to the ceiling and hold for a few seconds.
4. Release, then repeat three times.

The Throat Center

The most important part of the throat center is the production of sounds. The purpose of exercises for the throat area is to free the throat, tongue, and jaws, and to open the sinus and air passageways for free flow of movement so that self-expression comes easily and comfortably.

FISH POSE

1. Sit on the floor in a half-lotus position with your baby lying on his back on the floor horizontally in front of you.
2. Slip one hand under your baby's upper back and with your other hand gently hold your baby's legs in place.
3. Then gently lift the baby's chest up off the floor a few inches so that his neck can stretch back and his head drops down to touch the floor. This is a way to release the neck from its habitual incline forward.
4. Hold this pose for ten seconds, then release. Repeat the movement five times. Be very careful with your baby's neck—move it slowly and easily. If your baby is uncomfortable, raise the baby's chest a shorter distance from the floor.

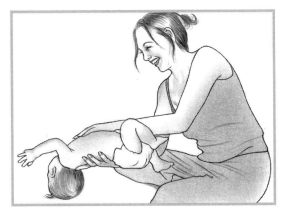

FISH POSE

IMITATION OF SOUNDS

1. Cradle your baby in your arms so you can see her face.
2. As your baby makes sounds, copy her sounds back to her and let her hear what her vocalizations sound like. To encourage imitation, make sure you are face-to-face with her so that she can see your facial expressions and mouth movements.
3. Repeat this as many times as she finds enjoyable.
4. Eventually try to get her to imitate your sounds. When she does imitate, repeat her repetition and smile in encouragement.

The Head Center

The purpose of the movements in the head center is to begin to activate the eyes so that your baby is visually absorbing all the information needed to live in the world. Your baby's eyes should work together to process this information. The head center requires that your baby understand that objects continue to exist even when he no longer sees them. Babies enjoy games, like peek-a-boo, that demonstrate object permanence.

MODIFIED BRIDGE POSITION

1. Sit on your heels with your baby sitting on his heels in front of you and facing outward.
2. Hold your baby's feet and pull his hands back behind him.
3. Encourage him to hold his feet. Try to help him lean back until his elbows touch the floor.
4. Reach one hand under your baby's buttocks to gently lift them off his heels while you anchor your baby's feet with your other hand. This will stretch out his spine and help him form the beginning of a back bend. At this point, the baby will no longer be able to hold

his feet, but his hands and arms will move out to the sides. His head, neck, and upper back will still be in contact with the floor. If this proves too difficult, you can support his full weight in this position by lifting him off the floor.

5. Hold this position for ten seconds, then release the buttocks down gently.

6. Repeat this pose five times.

SWAN POSE

1. First, set your baby in the Cobra position (see page 122).

2. Kneel behind your baby as he lies on the floor on his stomach. Tuck your feet under your buttocks and curl your toes toward the floor.

3. Place both of your hands at your baby's sides.

4. Slide your hands forward under his armpits; continue to slide them forward until your elbows touch the floor and your forearms are up off the floor facing away from you.

5. Turn your palms to face each other and hold your baby's head between them.

6. Rock back toward your heels slightly, keeping your elbows on the floor while lifting the baby's head, arms, and shoulders up off the floor. The torso should lift a couple of inches while the rest of his body remains on the floor.

7. Pause for a few seconds as your baby gets a chance to look around, then lower him down.

8. Repeat this five times to open up the entire throat and chest area.

9. Next, as you lift up his head with your hands, lift his hands and arms straight out to the sides, perpendicular to the body, as if he is about to fly away.

10. Hold for a ten seconds, release, and repeat five times.

PEEK-A-BOO

You can hide or you can hide your baby, but in either case, the delight of shouting "Peek-a-boo" when one of you is "found" should be unbounded.

The Crown Center

The purpose of the movements in the crown center is to stimulate the top of the head, bringing energy into the brain to stimulate the connection to the Higher. For the crown center, headstands are beneficial since they allow the blood to flow easily to the brain. This oxygenates the brain and the upper endocrine glands.

Be sure to make these exercises fun. Offer treats for reinforcement and use a few toys for motivation. Remember that at this age it is too early to expect your baby to imitate a position you demonstrate. Babies do not really imitate easily until they are close to two years of age.

HEAD STAND

1. Lay your baby flat on her back on the floor with her feet toward you while you stand above her facing her. BE CAREFUL.
2. Bend your knees if necessary and lean over to lift her legs and hips off the floor. Continue lifting her lower body up and toward you while letting her head maintain contact with the floor.
3. Lift until she is in a near vertical position with her feet pointing up toward the ceiling. For safety, *make sure you are supporting all of the baby's weight* so that she is resting very softly on the top of her head.

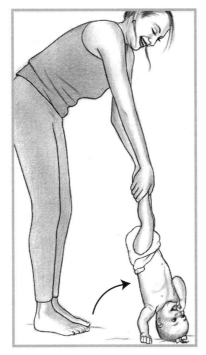

HEAD STAND

4. Hold this position for five seconds before gently releasing her body away from you and back down to the floor. Be extremely careful not to harm her neck during the release.

5. Repeat five times.

Note: Be sure to support her back where needed with one hand under her buttocks or back.

BREATHING

1. For a fun way to begin to stimulate your baby's breathing, try nose blowing to release the air from the lungs.
2. Using a tissue, show your baby how to blow about five to ten short breaths to empty the lungs and allow fresh air to move fully and fill the lungs.
3. Give him a chance to copy your movements.
4. Do this five times.

CHILD'S POSE

Between movements, it's a good idea for you and your baby to partake in a resting position called Child's Pose. During this posture, try the standard version while your baby performs a more modified format, since his little body does not have the same proportions as your adult body.

For your Child's Pose:

1. Sit on your heels with your legs together and lean forward, rounding down over your knees and letting the top of your forehead rest on the floor.
2. Drape your arms along the sides of your legs down to your feet.
3. Rest for a few seconds until you feel like sitting back up.

To modify this posture for your baby:

1. Have your baby sit on his heels and help him round over forward while opening his knees to the sides.
2. Let his forehead touch the floor while his arms are stretched straight out along his sides and touching the floor.
3. Allow him to rest as long as he feels comfortable in this position.

At this stage of your baby's development, you probably get most of your exercise chasing him around. In a quiet moment, feel free to assume your crossed-leg positions and stretch out as indicated on pages 53 to 55. Also feel free to do a Downward Dog:

1. Stand straight up with your legs at hip width apart and feet flat on the floor.
2. With a straight back, lean over to the floor, placing your hands flat on the floor with your fingers stretched and spread apart; do not twist the wrists.
3. Stretch up to the ceiling from the buttocks with the legs lengthened and the back and arms straight and lengthened so that your body forms a V shape.
4. If possible, gently push heels flat against the floor to increase the stretch in the back of the legs.
5. Hold for several minutes, then release down to place knees on the floor.
6. When rested, resume the position and hold for a few more minutes. Repeat three times.

Organizing Your Own Yoga Baby Club

A wonderful way to continue the Yoga Baby program once you and your baby have completed the first ten sessions is to form a local Yoga Baby club. A Yoga Baby club allows you to experience the process of learning intuitive parenting together, share your experiences with others, and educate yourselves about ongoing parenting issues. Many parents feel quite isolated and unable to find a way to readily connect with other mothers and fathers going through the same process. I suggest getting together with new parents from your neighborhood or from parenting classes. There are many such programs around the country, usually affiliated with local hospitals or with your local YWCA. These are excellent starting points for assembling like-minded parents.

Select a group of parents with babies roughly about the same age. The idea is not to compare whose baby does what the soonest; that is a waste of time. Instead, try to find ways to bond with your babies as your babies develop.

I have given you the beginning tools, and now it is up to you to continue with them. A parents' group is an excellent way to continue this. You may want to invite a professional such as a pediatrician, a child development specialist, or a preschool educator to some of your meetings. Although this is not essential, it may add a fresh perspective to the group.

AGENDA

Try to keep to a no-frills, down-to-business approach to your Yoga Baby club meetings. It is important to keep the focus as child-centered as possible. Remember, your goal is to find ways to parent intuitively and to bond with your baby. Encourage parents to share their deeply held feelings, such as being frightened or feeling stupid or inadequate. It is also important to allow for ambivalent or even hostile feelings about being a parent. Encourage the positive, but remember that clearing the air about some negative feelings—without dwelling on them—is a positive step forward.

Decide on an order to your meetings. It's beneficial to get business done first and then indulge in some hands-on Yoga Baby work to experience quality time with your baby and new friends. Decide which monthly periodicals and newsletters are of benefit to the group and be sure everyone gets a copy of relevant material. First and foremost, experience the joy of parenting, share the frustration of it with others, and seek out knowledge.

EDUCATION

Part of the purpose of the club is to educate yourselves, so pick several topics about which all of you have concerns and decide who will be doing research on the books to be read or the experts to be consulted. These are tasks that can be assigned and shared so that everyone benefits from the learning process.

Here are some suggestions for topics to discuss at your Yoga Baby club meetings:

1. The value of therapeutic touch
2. Stages of child development
3. Bedtime battles
4. Discipline
5. Toilet training
6. Developing creativity
7. How to influence children
8. How to listen and talk to children
9. Encopresis/Enuresis
10. Common medical conditions
11. CPR training for parents of babies

LOCATION

If you rotate the location of your Yoga Baby club each time you meet, no one person will be overwhelmed by the task. As discussed earlier in the book, make sure the area where yoga sessions will be done is clean and hygienic. A quiet, dimly lit spot is best. If the floor is not carpeted, have padded mats available. Enhance the ambiance of the room by adding scents, music, and colors that pertain to your session.

LEADERS

It will take one or two highly motivated parents to take charge of organizing and assembling the group. This will help keep the group from falling apart. Groups have a life of their own, but they do require a solid energy base. In assembling the charter members of the group, look for men and women who have a variety of experience to bring to the group and who have demonstrated competence in some aspect of group skills, whether as part of a volunteer organization or a neighborhood alliance or in running a large family. These members will then be accustomed to the work involved in making something happen.

RULES

Each club has to have a few rules. In a club that meets once a week, one rule might be that those who are enrolled must not cancel more than three times in a six-month period or they cannot be part of the club. The consistent involvement of club members demonstrates commitment. Just as babies require stability and consistency, so does a club.

FIRST YEAR

The first year of a new club is always the trickiest and will determine if the club lasts or not. Once you begin your club, do not admit new members until you feel comfortable with the parents and babies who are already participating. This way, you will have less disruption and will enhance the possibility of developing some group cohesion. Remember that you will be developing relationships with other parents that may last a very long time; there are bound to be some shaky times as people get to know each other and begin to accept each other's quirks.

NEW MEMBERS

After the first year, it's a good idea to seek new members at a predetermined time (for example, the month of September each year) so that you can interview new members and admit them in an orderly fashion without disrupting the achievements of the already established group. Devise rules about how you select and admit members and determine who will make the decision about admitting new members so that everyone feels included in the process.

I hope you have enjoyed your ten sessions of Yoga Baby and that you have come to know the unique nature of your baby. I wish all new parents the best as they continue to develop the intuitive parenting skills that will allow them to be the best parents possible. Remember, you are nurturing a rising star for the next millennium—Good luck!

Yoga Classes and Resources

ARKANSAS
Barefoot Studio
3604 Kavanaugh Rd.
Little Rock, AR 72205
(501) 661-8005

ARIZONA
The Path Center for Hiking,
Yoga, and Meditation
P.O. Box 3933
Sedona, AZ 86340
(877) 999-PATH or
(520) 282-7223
(520) 282-7331 (fax)

CALIFORNIA
The Expanding Light Retreat
14618 Tyler Foote Rd.
Nevada City, CA 95959
(800) 346-5350
(916) 478-7518 (fax)

The Center for Yoga, L.A.
230½ N. Larchmont Blvd.
Los Angeles, CA 90004
(800) 334-YOGA

Bikram's Yoga College of India
8800 Wilshire Blvd, 2nd fl.
Beverly Hills, CA 90211
(310) 854-5800
(310) 854-6200 (fax)

Iyengar Yoga Institute
of San Francisco
2404 27th Ave.
San Francisco, CA 94116
(415) 753-0909
www.iyisf.com

Richard Miller, Ph.D.
Anahata Press
1111 Grandview Road
Sebastapol, CA 95472
(415) 456-3909

Tim Miller
Ashtanga Yoga Center
118 West E Street
Encinitas, CA 92024
(760) 632-7093

Mount Madonna Center
445 Summit Rd.
Watsonville, CA 95076
(408) 847-0406
programs@mountmadonna.org

Yoga Journal
2054 University Ave.
Berkeley, CA 94704
(510) 841-9200
(510) 644-3101 (fax)
For subscriptions, books, and
tapes: 800-I-DO-YOGA

The Yoga Studio
650 E. Blithedale Ave.
Mill Valley, CA 94941
(415) 380-8800

COLORADO
Colorado School of Yoga
2162 E. Colorado Blvd.
Denver, CO 80222
(303) 758-4814

Rocky Mountain Institute
of Yoga and Ayurveda
P.O. Box 1091
Boulder, CO 80306
(303) 443-6923

Shoshoni Yoga Retreat
P.O. Box 410
Rollinsville, CO 80474
(303) 642-0116
www.shoshoni.org

HAWAII
The Maui School of
Yoga Therapy
1030 E. Kuiaha Road
Haiku, HI 96708
(808) 572-1414
(808) 572-5775 (fax)

Mana Le'a Gardens
(800) 233-6467
www.maui.net/~mlg

IDAHO
The Ashram
1574 Shaw Mountain Rd.
Boise, ID 83712
(208) 385-9475 or
(800) 858-YOGA
www.yogaville.org

ILLINOIS
Integral Yoga
595 Wicklow Ct.
Deerfield, IL 60015
(847) 317-9642
(800) 858-YOGA
www.yogaville.org

Sivananda Yoga Vedanta Center
1246 W. Bryn Mawr
Chicago, IL 60660
(773) 878-7771 or
(800) 783-9642
(773) 878-7527 (fax)

MASSACHUSETTS
Cape Ann Yoga Center
48 Blackburn Center
Gloucester, MA 01930
(978) 282-4567

Kripalu Center for
Yoga and Health
P.O. Box 793
Lenox, MA 01240
(413) 448-3400 or
(800) 741-SELF
www.kripalu.org

Phoenix Rising Yoga Therapy
P.O. Box 819
Housatonic, MA 01236
(413) 274-3515
www.pryt.com
Also located in CA, CT, FL,
GA, IL, KY, MD, MI, MN,
NY, NC, OH, PA, SC

NEW MEXICO
Ayurvedic Institute
1131 Menaul NE
Albuquerque, NM 87112
(505) 291-9698

International Kundalini Yoga
Teachers Association
Route 2, Box 4, Shady Lane
Espanola, NM 87532
(505) 753-0423
(505) 753-5982 (fax)

NEW YORK
Ashtanga Yoga Institute
325 East 41st St., #203
New York, NY 10017
(212) 661-2895

Equinox
140 East 63rd Street
New York, NY 10021
(212) 750-4900

OM Yoga Center
135 West 14th St., 2nd fl.
New York, NY 10011
(212) 229-0267
www.omyoga.com

Sivananda Yoga Vedanta Center
243 West 24th Street
New York, NY 10011
(212) 255-4560 or
(800) 783-YOGA
(212)727-7392 (fax)
www.sivananda.org

Yoga Zone
160 East 56th Street
New York, NY 10022
(212) 935-9642

TEXAS
Integral Yoga
4307 North Westberry Bridge
San Antonio, TX 78228
(210) 434-1738
(800) 858-YOGA
www.yogaville.org

VIRGINIA
Satchidnanda Ashram
Route 1
Buckingham, VA 23921
(800) 858-YOGA
(804) 969-3121
www.yogaville.org

WASHINGTON
Integral Yoga
7651 South Scatchethead Rd.
Clinton, WA 98236
(360) 579-3735
(800) 858-YOGA
www.yogaville.org

Bibliography

Ansari, Mark, and Liz Lark. *Yoga for Beginners*. New York: Harper Perennial, 1998.

Behavioral-Developmental Initiatives. *The Carey Temperament Scales*. Scottsdale, AZ, 1996.

Biziou, Barbara. *The Joy of Ritual*. New York: Golden Books, 1999.

Dukes, Sir Paul. *The Yoga of Healthy, Youth, and Joy*. New York: Harper and Brothers, 1960.

Ferber, Richard. *Solve Your Child's Sleep Problems*. New York: Simon and Schuster, 1985.

Goleman, Daniel. *Emotional Intelligence*. New York: Bantam Books, 1995.

Haas, Elson M. *Staying Healthy with the Seasons*. Berkely, CA: Celestial Arts, 1981.

Hittleman, Richard. *Richard Hittleman's Yoga 28-Day Exercise Plan*. New York: Bantam Books, 1970.

Judith, Anodea. *Eastern Body Western Mind*. Berkeley, CA: Celestial Arts, 1996.

Leach, Penelope. *Your Baby and Child.* New York: Knopf, 1997.

Levy, Janine. *The Baby Exercise Book.* New York: Pantheon Books, 1973.

Ohashi, Wataru, with Mary Hoover. *Touch for Love: Shiatsu for Your Baby.* New York: Ballantine Books, 1985.

Ohashi, Wataru, with Mary Hoover. *Natural Childbirth: The Eastern Way.* New York: Ballantine, 1983.

Oki, Masahiro. *Zen Yoga Therapy.* Tokyo: Japan Publications, Inc., 1979.

Pilates, Joseph. *Return to Life.* Boston: The Christopher Publishing House, 1960.

Schneider, McClure Vimala. *Infant Massage.* New York: Bantam Books, 1982.

Sumar, Sonia. *Yoga for the Special Child.* Buckingham, VA: Special Yoga Publications, 1996.

Thomas, Alexander, Stella Chess, and Herbert Birch. *Temperament and Behavior Disorders in Children.* New York: New York University Press, 1969.

Tortora. *Principles of Human Anatomy.* New York: HarperCollins, 1992.

Ullman, Robert, and Judyth Reichenberg-Ullman. *Ritalin Free Kids.* Rocklin, CA: Prima Publishing, 1996.

Walker, Peter. *Baby Massage.* New York: St. Martin's Griffin, 1995.

Yamamoto, Shizuko. *Barefoot Shiatsu.* Tokyo: Japan Publications, Inc., 1979.

Index

About the Author

DeAnsin Goodson Parker, Ph.D., is one of the world's leading experts in child psychology and holistic wellness. Her extensive work led to her recent creation of the Yoga Baby program, which has captured the focus of the international wellness community.

Dr. Parker is currently the director of the Goodson Parker Wellness Center on Manhattan's Upper East Side. As a certified psychoanalyst, a licensed psychologist, a certified school psychologist, and a certified yoga instructor, Dr. Parker has received honors for her NIMH fellowship work at both the Children's Village in Dobbs Ferry, New York, and Columbia University. She also maintains a private practice.

Parker runs the Web site www.yogababy.com for parents around the world to participate in the Yoga Baby program. Here they can ask specific questions and stay informed about new materials, training programs, and Yoga Baby centers that are being developed.